Achieving Oral Health

/ERSITIES AT MEDWAY

Achieving Oral Health: The social context of dental care

Third edition

G. Kent PhD
Lecturer in Clinical Psychology
Department of Psychology
The University of Sheffield
Sheffield

R. Croucher PhD
Senior Lecturer in Dental Public Health
Department of Dental Public Health
St Bartholomew's and the Royal London School of
Medicine and Dentistry
London

wright

EDINBURGH LONDON NEW YORK OXFORD PHILADELPHA
ST LOUIS SYDNEY TORONTO

Wright
An imprint of Elsevier Science Limited
Robert Stevenson House,
1-3 Baxter's Place,
Leith Walk,
Edinburgh EH1 3AF

First published as The Psychology of Dental Care 1984
Second edition 1991
Third edition 1998
Reprinted 1999, 2001
Transferred to digital printing 2002

British Library Cataloguing in Publication Data
A catalogue record for this book is available from the British Library.

ISBN 0 8236 1057 6

ELSEVIER
SCIENCE
your source for books,
journals and multimedia
in the health sciences
www.elsevierhealth.com

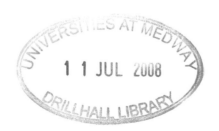

Typeset by Bath Typesetting, Bath

Contents

Foreword

Achieving Oral Health by Kent and Croucher, which has previously
been available as *The Psychology of Dental Care* in two very successful
editions, represents a further significant milestone on the road to total
acceptance of psychology and sociology as proper and ongoing
concerns of the dentist and the other members of a dental team as
they endeavour to provide high standards of oral and dental care.

The conception of 'The Dentist' has changed rapidly over the past
decades. Many progressive ideas have been added to the traditional
one that the dentist is a 'lone operator', a professional who is
narrowly constrained to techniques of mechanistic ablation and
repair. More progressive notions, such as 'The Biological Dentist',
'The Dental Team Leader', 'The Oral Physician' and, influentially,
'The Dentist as a Critical and Constructive Thinker', have been
proposed. Although some sharp debate has been occasioned by these
ideas, all the qualities implied in these notions are needed by the
modern dentist. Such a combination of abilities is reflected in the
General Dental Council publication *'The First Five Years – The
Undergraduate Dental Curriculum'*.

In the foreword to the second edition of this book, Sir David
Mason, then President of the General Dental Council, commended it
as a most suitable way of approaching an important subject area in
the manner required by the Council. For the reasons described above,
those wise sentiments can be fully endorsed with regard to this third
edition. It is a great pleasure for me to recommend this excellent text
to practitioners, students and all members of the dental team. As a
basis for raising standards of patient care, planning courses and
pointing to future developments, it will be of enormous assistance
and I am sure it will gain the extensive following achieved by its
predecessors.

Professor F. C. Smales

Acknowledgements

For their assistance in commenting on earlier drafts of various chapters, we would like to thank Mary Dalgleish, Rosie Croucher and Sharif Islam.

In addition to citations in the text, we would also like to thank the following for permission to reproduce material: Harcourt Brace Jovanovich for Fier M. (1980). Hypnosis in dentistry: a case history, *Dent. Surv.*, **56**, 12–13; Pergamon Press for Coe, W. C. (1980) Expectations, hypnosis and suggestion in behavioural change. In *Helping People Change* (F. H. Kanfer and A. P. Goldstein, eds); London; the American Academy of Oral Medicine for Jackson, E. (1975). Establishing rapport. 1. Verbal interaction. *J. Oral Med.*, **30**, 105–110; and CV Mosby for Hirsch, B., Levin, B. and Tiber, N. (1973). Effects of dentist authoritarianism on patient evaluation of dentures. *J. Prosthet. Dent.*, **30**, 745–748.

Chapter 1

Challenges for modern dentistry

Modern dentistry provides many challenges for the dental practitioner. Some of these involve the acquisition of technical skills, such as the ability to use new materials and provide new treatment options. While such skills form the foundation of dental care, technical expertise is always provided in a social context. Not only is there the relationship between dentist and patient, but also the interface between dentist and community and between the dentist and his or her team. The aim of this book is to provide the reader with some of the knowledge and skills, as they have been developed by sociologists and psychologists, that help dentists to work with greater success in this social context.

Achieving oral health

There are both opportunities and barriers to the achievement of oral health. First, there are changing trends in levels of oral disease. Overall, there has been a substantial improvement in the oral health of young people in the industrialized countries of the world. One important challenge involves the maintenance of these improvements into adulthood (Murray and Pitts, 1996). This general improvement can, however, mask variations due to geographic region and social class background. Not everyone has benefited to the same extent, and people from non-Western cultural backgrounds can be at particular risk. The challenge of worsening levels of oral disease in parts of non-industrialized countries has to be faced (Hobdell, 1996). Can the dental profession help to improve the oral health of all members of all societies?

As the demographic profile of industrialized countries changes to reflect the growing number of older people, new demands for different types of expertise in dentistry are being created. Will the need for the care of the common oral diseases by dentists diminish in some parts of the world? And could dentists be replaced by dental auxiliaries in many instances?

The extent to which improvements in oral health are due to clinical practice is debatable. Some argue that oral health is improving because of changes in society, rather than being due to improved professional care (Nadanovsky and Sheiham, 1994). Perhaps a reduction in the number of trained dentists will have relatively little impact on oral health. There are also debates as to whether the provision of information to patients about the prevention of dental disease can be effective in helping them to change their behaviour. Those involved in health promotion recognize that providing clinical services is only one part of a more broadly based exercise which will include working with schools, community groups, industry and supermarkets. Health promotion will involve arguing policies that involve preventive measures for achieving oral health, such as water fluoridation (World Health Organization, 1984). These obviously take place beyond the surgery. Does the dentist have a part in these activities and, if so, what should it be?

There are many interpersonal challenges. To treat disease successfully requires the development of special communication skills, such as an ability to provide reassurance, personal care and comfort. Successful cure offers an opportunity to improve the quality of life of individuals using high-quality restorative materials. In all of these instances, patient satisfaction with treatment is a crucial aspect of care.

The public is being encouraged to have a voice in the planning of local services and to make its views known as consumers of health care (Burke and Croucher, 1996). The need to overcome barriers to the receipt of dental care and to reduce anxiety and discomfort to an acceptable level remains.

The skills of dental practice

Making a realistic response to these different challenges means that the members of a dental team need to develop a wide range of knowledge, skills and ways of thinking (Croucher and Bradnock, 1995). These skills can be grouped under the following headings:

Clinical: The ability to recognize disease, interpret diagnostic tests, and formulate diagnoses and treatment plans.

Technical: The ability to employ those technical procedures necessary to treat oral disease.

Scientific: The ability to understand scientific principles and to apply them in dental practice; the ability to evaluate knowledge concerning the causes of disease and the benefits derived from the technologies used to treat oral disease.

Interpersonal: The ability to understand and communicate with people, influence their behaviour through communication and education, and form relationships with patients that enhance therapeutic outcomes.

Management: The ability to act as a manager of a small organization, in order to direct, coordinate and lead a dental team.

Ethical: The ability to understand the principles of ethical conduct and the ability to apply them appropriately in the context of dental practice.

Political advocacy: The ability to help groups and communities recognize their own health needs and goals, and to organize to achieve them.

Aims of the book

The main aim of this book is to help the reader to develop a foundation of sociological and psychological knowledge and skills as they relate to the achievement of oral health. It does this by introducing some of the key current debates within these disciplines. Applying knowledge from these subjects will help the reader to develop a clearer understanding of the opportunities and barriers that arise in achieving this goal. Psychology and sociology offer much to help members of the dental team to develop their work both in the dental practice and, if they choose, in the wider community.

The book presents certain principles which will apply in many settings, even though every situation may appear unique. Understanding these principles involves not only reviewing the results of research, but also examining some of the difficulties in making sense of the results. This background is important because it is not possible to write a 'how to do it' manual that would be applicable to all situations. Rather, the opportunity is created to recognize and apply the principles when these could be helpful.

The reader is provided with the foundations for a working knowledge of how sociology and psychology can be applied in daily clinical practice. This book aims to assist members of the dental team in making their occupation as rewarding and enjoyable as possible. Dentistry can be a stressful occupation, requiring a wide variety of abilities. Developing these abilities will help students to see those situations where patients complain or are uncooperative as challenges that can be resolved successfully.

Definitions of sociology and psychology

Sociology and psychology are two subjects that have a contribution to make to the development of the wider range of knowledge, skills and ways of thinking that are necessary for achieving oral health. Both psychologists and sociologists have a shared aim, which is to understand people's behaviour. Both are also concerned with social factors and how these come to exert their influence on behaviour.

Sociologists are interested mainly in the social and political organization of societies and how behaviour is influenced by the community in which a person lives. Variation can be identified by factors such as social class, religion, sex or age. Such influences include such large-scale factors as government policy towards funding the health services, allocation of resources between various specialities, and the beliefs held by people about health and illness. In the USA, for instance, about 8% of the Gross National Product is spent on health care, while in the UK about half this amount is spent. A person's socioeconomic status – whether he or she works in a highly paid professional job or a poorly paid manual one – is related to dental attendance patterns, dietary habits and the likelihood of developing oral disease. A sociologist is interested in not only how these differences are related to dental care but also their implications for health-promoting activity outside the surgery.

Psychologists, on the other hand, are more concerned with individuals and their personal relationships. The social context is still vitally important, but there is more emphasis on individuals and their reactions to their environment. For example, a psychologist might be interested in whether some patients expect and experience more pain than others, or how edentulousness can affect a person's self-esteem and willingness to engage in social activities. Some psychologists are interested in neurological mechanisms, but their main concern is with how these mechanisms affect behaviour. An individual may have a mental handicap due to a brain lesion, for example, and this becomes significant to a psychologist only when it affects the ability of that individual to function in society.

Sociology and psychology are therefore complementary subjects. Just as an anatomist will concentrate on the structural aspects of the body and a physiologist will be more concerned with biological processes, to gain a full understanding of one subject requires an understanding of the other. Both sociological and psychological viewpoints are necessary for an understanding of how people behave.

Evidence-based practice: are sociology and psychology only common sense?

Some may argue that the ideas and research reported in the chapters that follow are obvious to everyone. 'Common sense' is often used to make judgements in our daily lives. These judgements are often 'automatic', in the sense that little thought may be given to them. However, any process of reasoning behind common sense is implicit: it cannot be examined by others. The practice of science – whether social or clinical science – requires that an explicit process of reasoning is demonstrated.

The use of common sense in dentistry is commonplace. It has been noted that much dental activity is not based on reliable evidence and that there is limited evidence of positive outcomes for some treatments. The continued, 'common-sense', use of some treatments costs money: it has been estimated that if the evidence regarding wisdom tooth extractions was put into practice, many fewer extractions would be performed. This has important ethical and financial implications. There might be not only a reduction in patients' physical discomfort, but also a current annual saving of £800 000 in the UK (Richards et al., 1997). More challengingly, there is also evidence that some treatments have negative health outcomes. The indiscriminate use of some types of radiograph and some treatments for temporomandibular joint dysfunction are examples of the sometimes inappropriate and damaging use of interventions.

The pressures on health care spending means that, increasingly, there are demands for explicit judgements to be made about the effectiveness of different activities. Doing what has always been thought of as common sense is no longer enough. Financial support will be available for what can be shown to be effective, and in what circumstances.

Sociology and psychology contribute to evidence-based practice. Both are involved in examining and questioning what might have come to be accepted by many as common sense. They contribute to the ongoing general debate within dentistry as to what will work and what will not. Also, the application of their findings will enable the dental profession to develop a much wider role, involving more than enhanced clinical skills. This contribution will be described in the chapters that follow.

References

Burke, L. and Croucher, R. (1996). Criteria of good dental practice generated by general dental practitioners and patients. *Int. Dent. J.*, **46**, 3–9.

Croucher, R. and Bradnock, G. (1995). The behavioural sciences in the undergraduate curriculum: which department should teach them? *Community Dent. Health*, **12**, 125–127.

Hobdell, M. (1996). Delivery of oral health care and implications for future planning:

developing countries. In *Community Oral Health* (C. Pine, ed.) pp. 298–306, Oxford: Wright.

Murray, J. J. and Pitts, N. (1996). Trends in oral health. In *Community Oral Health* (C. Pine, ed.) pp. 126–146, Oxford: Wright.

Nadanovsky, P. and Sheiham, A. (1994). The relative contribution of dental services to the changes and geographical variations in caries of 5 and 12 year old children in England and Wales in the 1980s. *Community Dent. Health*, **11**, 215–223.

Richards, D., Lawrence, A. and Sackett, D. L. (1997). Bringing an evidence-base to dentistry. *Community Dent. Health*, **14**, 63–65.

World Health Organization (1984). *Health Promotion. A Discussion Document on the Concept and Principles.* Copenhagen: World Health Organization Regional Office for Europe.

Chapter 2

The social context of oral health

In this chapter, we review the definitions of health that are used by lay and professional people. Dentists and patients often have very different views of what is meant by good oral health. We also examine current measures of oral health and the contribution that socio-dental indicators can make in developing a broader perspective to measurement. Third, the factors that have been identified as determining oral health are described. Finally, the implications for the development of oral health education and promotion policy are considered.

Definitions of health

Two broad definitions of health can be identified. First, there is that involving biophysical wholeness. This approach involves identifying biological disturbances or ruling out the presence of disease by recording its absence. Disease is determined by medically defined abnormalities in anatomical structures or in physiological or biochemical processes. The aim is to identify any pathological abnormality diagnosed by signs that signify the existence of a pathological lesion, such as caries. This definition makes a clinician into a kind of detective who responds to the symptoms reported by his or her patients. This approach to defining health also assumes that symptoms are used by a patient as a cue for accessing health services. As will be shown in the next chapter, this is not always the case.

An alternative definition of health has been presented by the World Health Organization (1948, 1984), which defined health as being different from the absence of disease, rather a state of complete physical, mental and social well-being. This definition has been welcomed as providing a positive perspective to health, with an emphasis upon social context and well-being. It also presents a holistic definition, including within it not only physical and psychological aspects but also the ability to make and develop social relationships. This definition also implies a concern for function, since it implies that health involves the individual being able to take part in his or her normal social roles, such as parenting and going to work. The importance of this holistic perspective for defining and measuring oral health will be outlined later in this chapter.

On the other hand, this World Health Organization definition has been criticized for proposing an unattainable ideal which cannot be measured easily. A positive definition of health implies a process of continuous adaptation rather than the achievement of a static state. Second, it assumes that there is a consensus within society as to what health is. However, many studies have shown that people vary in their subjective assessments of symptoms. What constitutes health for one person may not constitute health for another.

Thus, the disease model of health concentrates on the reduction of disease, while the World Health Organization's definition is more oriented to the achievement of physical, social and psychological well-being. This difference is of more than just academic interest, since it highlights a fundamental issue for dental health professionals. Should the main aim of a dentist be just to reduce disease and make people dentally fit or should the aim be to increase patients' social and psychological well-being? Does one aim exclude the other?

What ideas about health do people have?

Studies of different groups within the population have shown that there is considerable variation in ideas about health. The French people involved in one of the first studies on this topic used three ideas: the absence of disease (described as 'health in a vacuum'); being able to resist or cope with illness ('reserves of health'); and the complete state of holistic well-being ('equilibrium'), which was rarely attainable (Herzlich, 1973). These ideas have been noted in other studies, although the terminology may vary. Williams (1983) identified the ideas of absence of disease, balancing strength and weakness and being able to take part in normal life (a functional definition) in a sample of older Scottish people.

Other studies have also demonstrated variations between different social groups. d'Houtard and Field (1984) found that respondents in professional and clerical occupations had positive ideas about health (i.e. their definition corresponded with the World Health Organization approach), whilst respondents in manual occupations used more negative ideas, tending to define health as the absence of disease. This difference might reflect social background, as respondents with more years of formal education might have more ability to develop abstract ideas about health. Women are more likely than men to use functional ideas, such as being able to carry out all their activities, both within and outside the home (Blaxter and Paterson, 1982; Pill and Stott, 1982; Cornwell, 1984). Perhaps the different social responsibilities of everyday life that women and men need to deal with lead to different types of responses to symptoms.

The studies reported above were mostly conducted with small groups of people. A much larger sample was involved in a later study by Blaxter (1990). She found that there was little variation between respondents, who generally tended to choose the idea of 'absence of disease', with the following exceptions:

- Young men were more likely to view health in terms of physical strength and fitness whilst young women were more likely to answer in terms of energy, vitality and ability to cope.
- Middle-aged respondents viewed health in terms of mental well-being and contentment.
- Women were more likely to include good social relationships in their answers.

Ideas about health in other cultures

Ethnic minorities are groups with a long shared distinguishing history, with features such as common geographical origin, religion, language and literature (Hopkins and Bahl, 1993). Howlett et al. (1992) examined Blaxter's data further to compare the health beliefs of members of ethnic minorities. Compared with White respondents, Asians were more likely to define health functionally, whilst Afro-Caribbeans were more likely to reply in terms of energy and physical strength. Illness was generally attributed to bad luck by these ethnic minorities.

Many ethnic groups, while incorporating certain elements of scientifically based understanding of disease and illness into their lives, also adhere to more traditional and divergent ideas about health and illness. These associated health beliefs and behaviours are sometimes called folk beliefs. Older women, who are often more steeply versed in traditional health beliefs than men and who often act as the first line of health advice within the family, may adopt a combination of scientific and folk traditions to attempt to treat illness. This complementary approach is not necessarily harmful. Many folk treatments (which may include specific ritual behaviours, and the use of teas and other folk remedies) may, from a strictly medical standpoint, be viewed as unproved or ineffective but are seen as playing a highly positive role in terms of psychological well-being. Folk treatments allow an individual to address the social imbalances that are considered significant in causing a particular condition within the ethnic tradition (Hopper, 1993).

An appreciation of the cultural meanings of health and disease is important in understanding why people accept or do not accept professional health care. One oral health example is provided by a study of the Hong Kong Chinese. In Hong Kong, major differences exist between traditional lay health concepts and professional ones. Traditional Chinese health beliefs comprise a balance between and interaction of Yin and Yang, the vital forces in both the universe and the body, as the basis for maintaining health. A disturbed equilibrium of vital forces will manifest itself as disease. Treatment involves attempts to restore the equilibrium, often through a range of dietary products. For example, according to this system of beliefs, gum disease results from too much fire in the stomach, and it is treated with a cooling herb tea.

Furthermore, an understanding of cultural background is important when attempting to change health beliefs and attitudes (Lee et al., 1993). Cheng (1990) reviewed the influence of cultural beliefs of individuals, families and society on the treatment of birth defects such as cleft lip and palate. He argues that it is important to understand these beliefs because studies have reported a higher incidence of cleft lip and/or palate among Asian/Pacific populations.

These ideas are extremely important to practitioners working in a multicultural society. Cultural beliefs about the sources of illness and correspondingly appropriate forms of treatment may be interpreted as providing a barrier to professional health care. Many members of ethnic minorities may lack familiarity with Western diagnostic techniques and treatments and thus be anxious about taking advantage of Western interventions. A person may delay seeking dental treatment from a dentist due to reliance on home remedies. This could reduce the effectiveness of any planned health education activities and dental services available for improving the oral health status of the community.

Health care providers' ignorance of cultures can also impair their communication with patients, resulting in culturally irrelevant services or misinterpretation of side-effects of folk medicines. Successful communication requires recognition and consideration of cultural diversity and differing communication styles. Dismissal of beliefs held by people from other cultures — termed *ethnocentrism* — can create a barrier of misunderstanding. Health professionals would benefit from a deeper understanding of cultural beliefs and practice, and an acknowledgement of respect for these practices. Developing this understanding of ethnic minority cultures by Western scientific medical practitioners and health care providers may also improve the use of health care services (Uba, 1992; Bahl, 1993).

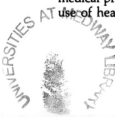

What is oral health?

Recent definitions of oral health are starting to reflect the ideas outlined earlier. They have become more holistic in their perspective and also seek to develop the links between oral health and general health, recognizing the complementary contribution that each makes to the other. These factors have been recognized in the following definition:

> Oral health is a standard of health of the oral and related tissues which enable an individual to eat, speak or socialise without active disease, discomfort or embarrassment and which contributes to general well-being. (Department of Health, 1994).

Measuring oral health

The ability of conventional measures of dental disease such as the Decayed, Missing and Filled Teeth index (DMFT) to measure all aspects of oral health is problematic. The DMFT is really a measure of dental history rather than of current dental health. A patient's teeth may be missing because of planned extractions due to overcrowding, may never have erupted or may have been lost because the patient had an accident.

Conventional dental measures such as the DMFT are based around professional judgements of the presence of disease, but there is a question about their reliability. The reliability of a measure is ascertained by asking at least two clinicians to examine patients independently. If both report the same results (i.e. they agree that a sign is either absent or present), then their measures are considered to be reliable. It is often assumed that all dentists would agree and come to the same conclusions when examining patients, but when this assumption has been put to the test some disconcerting results have arisen. For example, Smith (1977) asked two dentists to examine patients for signs of temporomandibular joint disorder. Smith found that there was total disagreement for 10% of the sample. For all the remaining patients, each dentist recorded many signs and symptoms not noted by the other.

We should also recognize that some oral conditions, such as malocclusion, are not diseases. As well as problems with interpretation and reliability, it has been argued that clinical assessments are too narrowly based, giving insufficient attention to the social consequences of oral conditions. The lay person, using psychological and social factors, should be able to supplement the professional perspective.

Furthermore, comparisons between clinical and functional criteria can be made. Often, the effects of a condition cannot be predicted by a knowledge of the severity of the impairment. This is shown most clearly by research on denture patients. Attempts have been made in several studies to relate clinical assessments of denture quality on such criteria as retention, fit, stability and bite force to patients' satisfaction with their appliances, but these have been largely unsuccessful. For example, Heyink et al. (1986) found only weak associations between dentists' and patients' appraisals of dentures. For the dentists, clinical indicators were most important, but for the patients, denture quality depended on how well they could function in practical everyday terms. Similarly, Haraldson et al. (1979) compared the bite forces of patients who were satisfied or dissatisfied with their dentures. No difference could be found. Although such studies indicate that extremely poor quality appliances are associated with the most dissatisfaction, the relationship is not a close one.

Impairment, disability and handicap

The World Health Organization (1980) has proposed that a distinction can be made between the objective pathology that a person may have and the disease's social and psychological effects. The term *impairment* could be used to refer to any physiological or anatomical loss or abnormality of structure or function. A broken leg, for example, is first of all an impairment. A fracture results in a *disability* because it imposes some sort of limitation on activity, for example, an inability to drive a car. Many individuals learn to live with their symptoms and come to an accommodation with the limitations imposed by disease. A third term is *handicap*. The broken leg can be a handicap when it makes it difficult for an individual to fulfil his or her roles in a family or society. In this way, two people could have similar impairments but not share a handicap: a broken leg would be very handicapping for a travelling salesman who relies on driving to make a living, but much less so for a writer for whom mobility is less important. Similarly, a person with a severe reading problem due to a brain lesion may be handicapped and disabled in our highly technological society but not in a culture where most communication is verbal rather than written.

Socio-dental indicators of oral health

Clinical measures concentrate on impairment while neglecting disability and handicap (Locker, 1988; Reisine, 1988). *Socio-dental indicators* measure the extent to which dental and oral disorders result in changes in behaviour and disrupt the ability to carry out everyday social roles. One of the first studies using this perspective was that of 254 elderly people living at home (Smith and Sheiham, 1979). Although this population described itself as in generally good health, three-quarters were edentulous. Having to wear dentures often caused pain and difficulties with chewing food, talking and singing. The authors noted that this sample's impairment (being edentulous) was the result of oral disease. One outcome of being edentulous was a limitation in function – chewing difficulty – which was disabling as it restricted the ability to eat. This was handicapping because respondents felt deterred from eating with others.

Measured in these ways, the effects of dental disease are widespread: Cushing et al. (1986) found that 26% of adults had experienced dental pain, 20% had difficulty with eating and 15% had had problems in communication during the previous year. Such discomfort can lead to high levels of disability or handicap for a patient. It is clear that some oral conditions, such as a disfiguring facial cleft, can have long-lasting and severe consequences on social and sexual relationships (Peter and Chinsky, 1974). So too can edentulousness. The wearing of dentures involves not only disabling problems such as the inability to chew certain foods but also a greater likelihood of mandibular dysfunctions such as headaches (Carlsson, 1976; Magnusson, 1980) and social problems such as refusing invitations to other people's homes and avoidance of speaking (Blomberg and Linquist, 1983). People may not need teeth to be adequately nourished, but they can be important if someone is to feel socially acceptable.

The ideas proposed by the World Health Organization have been used to develop scales, such as the Sickness Impact Profile (Bergner and Bobbit, 1981), which are designed to measure the effects of health difficulties on physical abilities (e.g. mobility, sleeping) and social roles (e.g. working relationships, recreation and communication). Comprehensive oral health assessment tools (Atchison and Dolan, 1990; Slade and Spencer, 1994; Leao and Sheiham, 1995) have also been developed. These measures are now recognized as providing better indicators of need than clinical measures alone, such as the DMFT, because they do not rely solely upon professional measures of disease but include the lay person's perspective. As such, they can be an important source of data for the planning and evaluating of dental services. At a more localized level, simpler measures of oral impacts have been developed which can be used by members of the primary health care team to encourage service uptake in older adults (Bush et al., 1996).

Variations in oral health

Epidemiology

Epidemiologists study the distribution and determinants of health-related conditions or events in populations. The results of epidemiology research can be used to plan interventions to control health problems. The determinants of these conditions can be genetic, environmental, biological or psychosocial. The concern of this text is social epidemiology, examining the environmental and psychosocial determinants of health.

Two basic epidemiological concepts are the prevalence (the number of people who have a disease) and the incidence (the number of new cases of a disease in a specified time period) of health problems. For example, the World Health Organization (1995) reviewed data on caries prevalence in 12-year-old children stored on its global data bank, gathered from 178 countries. This showed that 25% had very low levels of caries (a mean DMFT of 0.0–1.1), 42% had low levels of caries (a mean DMFT of 1.2–2.6), 30% had moderate levels of caries (a mean DMFT of 2.7–4.4), with the remainder having high or very high levels of caries (a mean DMFT greater than 4.5).

One example of using epidemiology to plan interventions arose from the observation that people living in certain areas had a lower prevalence of caries than those living in other areas. Variations in diet or behaviour were not apparent, and the cause was traced to naturally occurring fluoride in the water supplies of different communities. Identifying the important relationship between caries and fluoride led to the development of a range of topical and systemic strategies for fluoride use, which have made the most important recent contribution to the general improvement in oral health.

This section of the chapter will examine research on the relationship of ethnicity, age, sex and social class with oral health. This research has identified several important issues, including the need to target educational programmes for particular sections of the community.

Ethnic minorities

As most countries have become increasingly multicultural in their make-up, there has been a growing interest in identifying differences in oral health in different ethnic minorities. In the UK, for example, the dental health of ethnic communities does not reveal a consistent pattern. More caries are experienced among deciduous dentition, and there is variation in this among different ethnic groups (Prendergast et al., 1997) with, for example, higher levels of caries in young Asian children (Williams, 1984). Oral hygiene practices among five-year-old Asians are different from those of Caucasian children of a similar age (Williams and Fairpo, 1988), and marked differences in dentist visiting patterns among Bangladeshi and White children have been found: only 3% of White children had never visited a dentist compared with 30% of Bangladeshi children (Laher, 1990).

Bedi (1989) proposed that there are three distinct high-risk groups for young Asian children, depending upon their religion and English language competence. These differences, where levels of gross material deprivation are common to all communities, are linked to issues of culture and lifestyle which are potentially amenable to sensitively designed and meaningful health information. A study in Singapore also identified differences in both preventive knowledge and preventive dental behaviours among ethnic minorities. These were attributed to differences in education and exposure to product information (Soh, 1992).

Such patterns of disease could be due to many factors. The higher levels of caries may be due to dietary or weaning differences between ethnic and indigenous people, but they may also be due to a move from a culture in which little sugar is consumed to one where sugar consumption is higher.

Although these disease differences are marked, cultural variation can be given too much emphasis. In any society, patterns of disease and health care will vary quite dramatically among social groups. Many of the problems associated with minority status are in fact closely related to deprivation (Beal, 1990). Findings of cultural differences must be treated with caution, as immigrant status and the stress of adapting to a new culture can be important influences. Thus, when people seek health care or cope with symptoms in some other way, they may be influenced not only by cultural background but also by their new social environment (Hochstein et al., 1968; Douglass and Cole, 1979).

Sex

A useful distinction can be made between sex and gender (Oakley, 1993). The former refers to those elements of being male or female which are undeniably biological, whilst the latter to socially assigned meanings given to sexual differences. O'Mullane et al. (1993) note that, apart from tooth loss and edentulism, data on the relative levels of oral health of men and women are scarce. Evidence from Europe and to a lesser extent from the USA shows that women have fewer natural teeth than men and have higher levels of edentulism. In Europe there is some evidence that socially deprived rural women have the highest levels of edentulism. Data from the Republic of Ireland suggest that women working in the home have higher levels of tooth loss and edentulism than those working outside the home. Due to the lack of adequate detail in published reports, it is difficult to discern whether such differences in oral health are due to the availability, acceptability or accessibility of dental services. Women tend to attend for dental care more regularly than men, though there is some evidence that women are more fearful of dental treatment and also perceive cost as a barrier to dental care (Todd and Lader, 1991).

There is a need for further research to investigate why women tend to lose their natural teeth at an earlier age than men. It is apparently contradictory that women may attend more regularly but have a worse health status. It has been suggested in studies of medical care, where women consult the doctor more often but live longer, that the gender roles they have adopted have encouraged feelings of illness. An ability to provide social support and care has usually been perceived as a female characteristic. If women developed occupational and social roles similar to those of men, then there might be a diminishing of these gender and health differences, as the Irish data reported above suggest.

Age

Consideration of the relationship between age and oral health is important for two reasons. First, there is the concept of socialization, which is the term given to the process whereby we learn the values and norms of a group or society. It is an ongoing and gradual process which continues throughout life. By the age of three years, for example, children know many of the basic norms and conventions practised in their culture, such as the 'correct' toys for boys and girls and the occupations that adult males and females typically enter. Children are very adept at picking up such rules.

The process of transmitting general cultural information, including ideas about health, is termed *primary socialization*. MacEntee et al. (1991) suggest from their study of 521 people aged 70 years and over that the oral health and related behaviours established early in life are crucial. An interesting oral health example was provided by King (1978), who interviewed a group of mothers with young babies to establish the degree of comparison between mothers' and children's intakes of sugar. On a 24-hour basis, the average number of maternal sugar intakes was 4.7, whilst for their babies the average was 4.3. In addition, King noted that 61% of babies with a high sugar consumption also had mothers with a high sugar consumption. Her concern was that these early childhood habits, once learnt, would have a longer term impact upon the permanent dentition and possibly lead to obesity. The outcome of the parent acting as a role model for the child has also been demonstrated in adolescence by Astrom and Jakobsen (1996), who identified significant associations between parent and offspring oral health behaviours, such as tooth brushing and the drinking of sugar-free mineral water. Downer (1995) argues that children should be the number one priority in the development of dental services, so that the dental health of future adults can be safeguarded.

A second reason for being interested in the relationship between age and oral health is that older people often present particular oral health problems. Those who have always attended the dentist regularly will probably continue to do so and retain some or all of their teeth (Thomson and Cautley, 1996). One study investigated the oral health-related quality of life in 1242 older men (Kressin et al., 1996). Those with a higher oral health-related quality of life reported less dental pain or discomfort, fewer eating problems and less problem-based dental care utilization. Dental pain and oral discomfort were positively related to use of dental services. Slade and Spencer (1994) investigated the social impact of oral conditions in 1217 older people. Older age was associated with significantly greater amounts of impact, with edentulous males reporting higher impact scores than edentulous females. About 10% of this sample reported problems with chewing food and avoidance of certain foods fairly or very often. These impacts reflect a lifetime of disease experience.

Levels of dental anxiety may also vary by age. The Corah Dental Anxiety Scale was administered to a sample of 580 people aged between 50 and 89 years (Locker et al., 1991; Locker and Liddell, 1991), of which 8.4% were classified as dentally anxious, with older individuals having lower scores than the younger. An older dentally anxious person was less likely to have a source of regular dental care, less likely to have visited the dentist in the previous year and more likely to have avoided or delayed dental treatment.

Members of the primary dental care team should recognize that the general quality of life is clearly linked to oral health in older people. The dental condition may contribute to nutritional intake. Systemic diseases and the medications taken to treat them will also often have a direct effect on oral health, affecting salivary, oral motor and oral sensory function. It has been proposed that organisms of oral origin are responsible for systemic infection. This suggests a need for the development of alliances between primary oral and medical care teams, to ensure that any general health assessment of an older person includes an oral component, and that oral conditions, once identified, are treated.

Social class

Measuring social class

The measurement of social class has developed since the industrial revolution, when jobs became more differentiated than had been the case in farming-based communities (Abercrombie and Warde, 1988). The division of labour led to the development of classifications based on occupation, such as the Registrar General's classification. In this classification, all jobs are placed into one of six categories, each being assigned a social class. Social class I, for example, includes accountants, dentists, doctors and lawyers, whilst social class V includes labourers and office cleaners. These six categories can be collapsed into two: manual and non-manual. Whilst this method of classification has the advantages of being widely used and relatively simple, these are increasingly outweighed by disadvantages which limit the ability to fully explain inequality. Retired people, married women not in paid employment and unemployed people are excluded from the classification. Being a measure of individuals, it gives no indication of where groups with poor health are found. Finally, some people may not wish to divulge their employment status.

Table 2.1. Registrar General's social class classification

Social class	Description	Examples
I	Professional	Doctor, dentist
II	Intermediate	Manager, school teacher
IIINM	Skilled non-manual	Secretary, dental technician
IIIM	Skilled manual	Bus driver, carpenter
IV	Partly skilled	Postman, agricultural worker
V	Unskilled	Cleaner, labourer

Adapted from OPCS (1980).

Alternative, area-based measures are now being developed, which classify people according to the characteristics of the area in which they live. The classifications are developed using nationally collected census data (Jarman, 1984). When surveying the prevalence of disease in different areas, he not only assessed occupation but also the number of elderly people living alone, children aged under five years, one-parent families, and levels of unemployment and overcrowding. By taking this broader view, it was possible to delineate areas more accurately in terms of social background and deprivation. To classify an individual, only his or her address or postcode is needed, and this is usually easier to collect.

Several evaluations of these measures have been undertaken. Locker and Ford (1994) found that their area-based Canadian data had more advantages than disadvantages, compared with a household measure of income. They could identify small areas with high levels of health care needs, leading to better planning and the targeting of resources. This factor has been recognized by investigators in the UK, who have used an area-based measure, ACORN (A Classification Of Residential Neighbourhoods), to direct dental health promotion activities (Whittle and Davies, 1992). Locker and Ford (1994) also confirmed in their study that the environment has its own impact upon health. This argument had been proposed by other investigators (Blane, 1985; Davey-Smith et al., 1990). Low-income individuals living in a high-status area were found to have a better oral health status than their counterparts living in lower status areas.

Table 2.2. ACORN neighbourhood groups, allocated into three divisions with proportion of divisions within the UK (%)

Division		ACORN group	Proportion within the UK (%)
I	Modern family housing, higher incomes	B	
	Student and high-status non-family area	I	37.1
	Traditional high-status suburbia	J	
	Areas of elderly people	K	
II	Modern family housing for manual workers	A	20.9
	Older housing of intermediate status	C	
III	Very poor quality terraced housing	D	
	Urban local authority housing	F	33.9
	Low-income areas with immigrants	H	
	Unclassified	U	
IV	Rural areas	E	
	Housing with most overcrowding	G	8.4

Adapted from Sarll, Whittle & Mackie (1984).

Social class and oral health

There are many studies that demonstrate a relationship between social class health generally and oral health more specifically. In general, members of lower social classes in industrialized countries have a poorer dental health status, whether they are elderly English people (Steele et al., 1996), Brazilian nursery school children (Freire et al., 1996), Greek adolescents (Petridou et al., 1996) or English inner city preschool children (Holt et al., 1996). This relationship is reversed in non-industrialized countries, where it is the children with better educated and richer parents who have significantly more caries (Normark, 1993).

A UK study of 1658 children aged from 1.5 to 4.5 years demonstrated that dental decay was strongly related to social background (Moynihan and Holt, 1996). The challenging finding from such studies is that, even in situations where there are general reductions in dental disease being recorded for children, there is still a negative gradient between the different social classes. For example, Holt et al. (1996) compared data collected in 1966 and 1986. They concluded that over time there was little evidence of improvement in the dental health of young children, with a small proportion, mainly from the lowest social classes, suffering relatively severely from caries.

Table 2.3. A comparison of caries-free three-year-olds in 1973, 1981 and 1989 in a Hertfordshire town, related to social class (%)

Social class	1973	1981	1989
I	79	92	100
II	84	84	94
IIINM	71	89	88
IIIM	57	78	73
IV/V	49	71	71

Adapted from Silver, D. H. (1992).

This finding is reinforced by the work of Silver (1992), who examined three samples of three-year-old children over 16 years. Silver notes that the rate of caries reduction has decreased in recent years, with a slight deterioration being recorded in the lower social classes. Whilst nearly all the higher social class children were caries-free, less than three-quarters from the lower social classes were caries-free. A group of class-related practices was identified, with the lower social class families adopting less favourable behaviour. They were less likely to start tooth brushing at an early age or attend the dentist for check-ups, and more likely to use a comforter bottle for infants. Silver concludes that there is a need for the fluoridation of water supplies and an improvement in overall living conditions if further improvements in oral health are to take place in the lower social classes.

Explanations for social class differences

The Black Report (Blane, 1985) sought to understand why this gradient between health and social class exists. Four possible explanations for health inequalities were considered:

1. *The artefact explanation.* The results showing a relationship between social class and health are not really present in the community but are only due to the way data are collected. For example, reliance on death certificates may bias findings inappropriately. However, even when investigators have taken such problems into account, class differentials remain.

2. *The social selection explanation.* This proposes that health inequalities are created by a process whereby the healthy move up the social hierarchy and the less healthy move down. A person who is initially unhealthy may find it increasingly difficult to find skilled employment, and so may need to take on less and less well paid jobs. Conversely, a person who is healthy may find it relatively easy to gain higher educational qualifications, and so move up the social class scale. Whilst in general there are few data to support this explanation, in oral health it has been noted that schoolteachers rate the behaviour and personality of attractive children more highly and expect them to have higher academic achievements than their less attractive peers (Shaw et al., 1985). Perhaps having good oral health can improve a person's chances of obtaining a skilled position.

3. *The materialist explanation.* According to this explanation, inequalities in health have their origins in social and financial deprivation. Even though there has been an improvement in living standards, the lower social classes live in relatively more unhealthy environments, do more dangerous and insecure work, and have poorer housing and lower incomes. These factors are assumed to interact together, having a cumulative effect.

4. *Behavioural explanations.* These explain inequalities in terms of differences in knowledge and behaviour. Perhaps people from higher social classes have a greater appreciation of the role of diet and regular preventive care, and are more likely to act on this knowledge. This explanation has received much support, since such lifestyle differences have been shown to be involved in many diseases. People with higher social class parents are more knowledgeable about the causes of dental decay, for example (see Beal, 1983). Attwood et al. (1990) have suggested

that class differences in dental health are also influenced by the following lifestyle factors:

- Children from affluent areas are more likely to use fluoride toothpaste.
- The intake of refined carbohydrate is lower in the upper socio-economic groups.
- The parents from upper social class groups are more interested in oral health and seek advice and routine screening from a dentist more frequently.

Thomson et al. (1996) developed a child neglect scale. They studied the responses of the parents of nearly 300 Australian children aged 10–11 and 14–15 years. Dental neglect was greater amongst males, those whose mothers had less education and those for whom a parent's last dental visit was symptom-driven rather than for a routine examination. de Vries et al. (1990) investigated the relationship between caries prevalence and food intake in 284 Dutch schoolchildren. The children of less-educated parents were at an increased risk of 'unhealthy' food habits.

It has also been suggested that, in addition to these factors, members of the lower social classes are reluctant to undertake long-term planning for the future, whereas those in the higher social classes are more future-oriented. This orientation is perhaps a feature of industrialized societies, where job security and careers are more readily available to the higher social classes.

Which explanation is correct?
It seems likely that both materialist and behavioural explanations contribute to socioeconomic differences in oral health. Their contribution is thought to continue from childhood throughout adolescent and adult life. Sakki et al. (1994) established that issues of lifestyle, such as dietary habits, smoking and alcohol consumption and physical activity, were associated with decayed tooth surfaces in 780 Finnish adults, whilst Keogh and Linden (1991) demonstrated that higher social class adult respondents had clearer knowledge, more positive attitudes and more appropriate behaviour related to dental health than respondents from the lower social classes.

Although often found in combination (i.e. low income, cariogenic dietary habits and reduced access to dentists) and all part of general social deprivation, it is important to recognize that both material circumstances and behaviour have separate influences. This was illustrated by the work of Gratrix and Holloway (1994). They investigated oral health issues in two groups of urban primary schools: one group with the highest prevalence of dental caries; the other with the lowest prevalence of dental caries. The five-year-old children in the highest caries prevalence group came from communities that had high area deprivation scores. There were lower proportions of babies born of normal birthweight and a lower vaccination uptake. Their families were less likely to own a car, and the children were more likely to receive free school meals. Complementing these measures of social deprivation was a range of parental practices, primarily linked to infant feeding and weaning, which placed young children at greater risk. Similar findings were reported by Thomas and Startup (1992), who studied the dental health of 405 five-year-old schoolchildren living in rural Wales. Lower disease levels were positively associated with the household ownership of a telephone and a car and a higher maternal educational attainment. Car ownership may be used as an indicator of disposable income. The resources required to buy and run a car will be beyond people living at or below subsistence level. Car ownership allows a family to have mobility to access health care and supermarkets. We should also recognize that having a low income means that choosing a nutritionally adequate diet can be difficult to achieve.

The contribution of the dentist to achieving oral health

The focus of this chapter has been to describe ideas about health and the factors that determine health. One conclusion that can be drawn is that environmental issues are a major determinant of health, including oral health, and that these are complemented by a range of individual behaviour, attitudes and knowledge. We will now consider the implications of this conclusion for achieving oral health, and outline the possible contribution of dentists to this goal.

Changing patterns of disease

Most studies in industrialized countries have reported that the prevalence of caries has declined in recent years. Between 1973 and 1993 in the UK, there was a decline in caries experience of 55% in the deciduous teeth of five-year-old children, 75% in the permanent teeth of 12-year-olds and 74% in 14-year-olds (Downer, 1994). The prevalence of dental caries in developed countries in five and 12-year-old children has been shown to have decreased substantially, with increasing numbers being found to be caries-free (Murray, 1994).

Such results could be taken to indicate that the dental profession has had a substantial impact on the incidence of dental disease. Caries levels in the non-industrialized countries, where professional dental care is less available, are tending to increase considerably. The overall mean declines in caries that are reported also obscure variation within countries. Most of the dental caries are now found in a relatively small part of the child population. These children are often found in deprived and poor communities (Ellwood and O'Mullane, 1995).

It cannot necessarily be concluded, however, that it is the efforts of primary dental care teams that have resulted in the lower levels of oral disease reported above. There are two reasons to believe that professional dentistry has had only a relatively small impact on prevalence.

First, not everybody attends the dentist on a regular basis, whether to receive treatment or preventive advice about the use of fluoride. Reference has been made to the 'missing 50%' who the dentist rarely, if ever, sees (Murray, 1996). Although a great many people do not visit a dentist, the level of caries is nevertheless declining.

Second, the contribution of health services to health in general have been critically reviewed in an analysis by McKeown (1979). McKeown examined the evidence for the reasons for the improvement in health in the UK over the last 150 years. He concluded that the decline in mortality predated knowledge about the prevention or effective treatment of diseases such as tuberculosis, pneumonia and whooping cough. Three factors were identified as having the greatest impact upon improvements in health: better food; environmental improvement such as a quality water supply; and a reduction in average family size. Social factors, such as changes in economic and social conditions, were therefore of more importance than the health services.

McKeown's ideas have recently been applied to dental services. Nadanovsky and Sheiham (1994, 1995) have reviewed data from 18 industrialized countries, using information about dental caries, the presence of dental services and social factors such as the widespread availability of fluoridated toothpaste. Their findings suggest that availability of dental services was relatively unimportant in explaining the differences in dental caries in 12-year-olds in England and Wales. In 1989, 34% of the variation in the DMFT of five-year-old children was explained by dental service activity and 57% by social factors. For 12-year-old children in 1988, 29% of the variation in DMFT was explained by dental service activity and 46% by social factors. Whilst there may be disagreement about the precise contribution of these factors to oral health, it seems clear that further reductions in dental caries will be achieved if a broad perspective with respect to prevention is adopted and the primary dental care team learn from the experience of treating and preventing other diseases (Krasse, 1996).

Health promotion and health education

The recognition of the importance of the environment and structural issues to health has led to the development of health promotion programmes. Health promotion has been defined as the process of seeking to improve or protect health through a range of activity, including behavioural, socioeconomic and environmental policy change (World Health Organization, 1984). More specifically, the range of health promotion activities includes the following:

1. Health education. This includes giving information about health, offering advice and trying to encourage the development of personal self-confidence. Opportunities for this exist in group situations, such as schools, and dentist–patient contact. Radio, television or newspapers may also provide information and advice. The latter group is non-personal, however, and cannot be focused on an individual's specific needs.
2. Personal preventive health services, such as immunization or oral cancer screening, and positive health services, such as smoking cessation programmes. Special initiatives might be planned for those patients who are unable to access professional dental care, whether for reasons of anxiety or distance.
3. Environmental measures, such as making the physical environment more conducive to health. This might include designing buildings better to reduce the chance of dental trauma in children or the optimal adjustment of the fluoride content of water to prevent dental caries (Burt and Eklund, 1997). The adjustment of fluoride in public water supplies to the optimal level of one part per million has been shown to be an effective method of reducing dental decay.
4. Involving the community, either to develop local services or to form self-help or pressure groups.
5. Organizational development, involving the implementation of policies that promote the health of staff and their clients, such as providing no-smoking areas or healthy catering services.
6. Economic and regulatory activity. This might involve changing taxation to make products either more or less expensive or the development of a code of practice that may, for instance, control the advertising of health compromising products (Catford and Nutbeam, 1984).

The fundamental issue is to make the healthy choices easier (Milio, 1986). Health education is an important part of overall health promotion activity. Interventions may not have long-term accept-ability without public understanding of the reasoning behind them. On the other hand, knowing what a healthy diet should contain will not be very helpful to those people without the resources to purchase the diet, and will not affect the availability in shops of the products that constitute it.

Health promotion activity provides several difficult challenges for the dentist, whose training has usually been limited to the teaching of small groups or individuals in the dental surgery. Communication skills are an important asset to build upon, but they would need to be developed for use in activities such as lobbying for regulatory change or promoting water fluoridation. Additional skills would also be required, for example, in planning and implementing strategies, and identifying organizations and groups with whom these strategies can be implemented. There are several recent examples of the development of this range of activity. Doctors and pharmacists have been successfully encouraged to prescribe and dispense sugar-free paediatric medicine (Bentley et al., 1993), whilst health visitors have been involved in campaigns to improve dental registration for preschool children (Bentley and Holloway, 1993). Dental public health services in Toronto were successfully reorganized through the involvement of community groups in the review process (Lee, 1991).

The contribution of fluoride to changing caries levels

The previous section suggests that dentists can act as advocates, making a case for change on behalf of the communities within which they work. Water fluoridation has been introduced in communities through the involvement of dentists (Castle, 1987). The most commonly cited measures that have contributed to changing caries levels (Petersson and Bratthall, 1996) involve fluoride – especially the fluoridation of water supplies but also the increased use of fluoride toothpastes, tablets and gels, fluoride rinsing programmes and dietary fluoride supplements. Other reasons have been proposed such as an increased dental awareness among the population, decreases in sugar consumption and the greater availability of dental health education programmes.

Several studies have investigated whether the fluoridation of water supplies reduces the social class differences in caries experience outlined earlier. Carmichael et al. (1989) demonstrated that fluoridation was effective in all social class groupings, reducing, but not eliminating, social inequalities. In a follow-up study 18 years later, these findings were compared in the context of the overall reduction of caries that had taken place. It was concluded that poor social background still disadvantaged some younger (five-year-old) children (Evans et al., 1996). Among 15-year-old children, water fluoridation eradicated any social class gradient in dental disease (Murray et al., 1991).

Slade et al. (1996) have argued from Australian data, where there are low levels of caries in children, that exposure to water fluoridation leads to lower caries experience in both the primary and secondary dentition, that caries experience is related to the amount of time that an individual is exposed to water fluoridation (longer period of exposure, less caries experience) and that socially disadvantaged people still receive the most benefit from this public health measure. There are ethical issues to consider concerning the introduction and use of fluoride: these are reviewed in Chapter 9.

New roles for the primary care dentist?

In addition to these wider health promotion skills, other proposals have also been made for the activity of dentists who recognize the changing context of dental care (Mautsch and Sheiham, 1995). These include developing managerial skills as the leader of a primary dental care team, providing complex, high-quality treatment and a commitment to the continuing education of colleagues. Dentists who wish to become involved in the community by providing talks to groups would also benefit by improving their presentation skills (Leeds, 1988).

Summary

The concern of this chapter has been to outline some issues from the wider social context within which members of the primary dental care team work: ideas about what constitutes health differ between people; ideas which are being increasingly incorporated into the measurement of oral health. These innovative measurements assess wider issues in health, moving beyond clinical measures of disease. Variations in oral health between different groups of society have been described.

Explanations for these variations, especially in the context of social class, have been assessed. The implications of these explanations for achieving oral health have been described, especially in the context of the contribution that dentists can make to this. Whilst the evidence suggests that this contribution has been limited in the past, there are opportunities available for health-enhancing activity both inside and outside the dental surgery.

Practice implications

- Because most members of the population support a negative definition of health, i.e. the absence of disease, members of the primary dental care team face an important challenge. There is the risk that health may be seen by the public as something taken for granted, only to be thought about when symptoms interfere with daily life. The challenge would not be necessarily to give information but to develop a set of ideas about health so that people felt more positive.
- Studies show that the values of dentists may not correspond with those held by lay people. It is not simply a question of which group holds the 'right' or 'correct' beliefs. Rather, the values may be different, and such differences have many implications for the practice of dentistry. For example, a dentist who is working from only a clinical set of values about the importance of disease will miss the significance of the patient's point of view. A treatment plan, though clinically correct, may not be feasible because it is inconsistent with a patient's priorities and difficulties.
- Older people may present particular challenges for primary dental care because of the need to consider the impact of systemic disease upon oral health and the need to collaborate with primary medical care teams.
- Ill-health is not only a result of failings in the health service but is also linked to inequalities in income, education, housing and working conditions, which affect people throughout their lives.
- A wider range of skills is needed by dentists to tackle these issues of ill-health. In addition to providing high-quality restorative care and managing the other members of the primary dental care team, working with other people outside the surgery can help to secure and enhance current achievements in oral health.

References

Abercrombie, N. and Warde, A. (1988). *Contemporary British Society*. Oxford: Blackwell.
Astrom, A. N. and Jakobsen, R. (1996). The effect of parental dental health behaviour

on that of their adolescent offspring. *Acta Odontol. Scand.*, **54**, 235–241.

Atchison, K. A. and Dolan, T. A. (1990). Development of the Geriatric Oral Health Assessment Index. *J. Dent. Educ.*, **54**, 680–686.

Attwood, D., Salapata, J. and Blinkhorn, A. (1990). Comparison of the dental health of 12-year-old children living in Athens and Greece. *Int. Dent. J.*, **40**, 117–121.

Bahl, V. (1993). Access to health care for black and ethnic minority elderly people: general principles. In *Access to Health Care for People from Black and Ethnic Minorities* (A. Hopkins and V. Bahl, eds) pp. 93–98, London: Royal College of Physicians.

Beal, J. F. (1983). Social factors and preventive dentistry. In *The Prevention of Dental Disease* (J. J. Murray, ed.). Oxford: Oxford University Press.

Beal, J. F. (1990). The dental health of black and ethnic minority communities. *Community Dent. Health*, **7**, 121–122.

Bedi, R. (1989). Ethnic indicators of dental health for young Asian schoolchildren resident in areas of multiple deprivation. *Br. Dent. J.*, **166**, 331–334.

Bentley, E. M. and Holloway, P. J. (1993). An evaluation of the role of health visitors in encouraging dental attendance of infants. *Community Dent. Health*, **10**, 243–249.

Bentley, E. M., Mackie, I. C. and Fuller, S. S. (1993). Pharmacists and the 'smile for sugar-free medicines' campaign. *Pharm. J.*, **251**, 606–607.

Bergner, M. and Bobbit, B. (1981). The Sickness Impact Profile: development and final revision of a health status measure. *Med. Care*, **19**, 787–805.

Blane, D. (1985). An assessment of the Black report's explanations of health inequalities. *Sociology of Health and Illness*, **7**, 423–445.

Blaxter, M. (1990). *Health and Lifestyles*. London: Routledge.

Blaxter, M. and Paterson, L. (1982). *Mothers and Daughters: A Three Generation Study of Health Attitudes and Behaviour*. London: Heinemann.

Blomberg, S. and Linquist, L. (1983). Psychological reactions to edentulousness and treatment with jawbone-anchored bridges. Acta Psychiatr. Scand., **68**, 251–262.

Burt, B. A. and Eklund, S. A. (1997). Community based strategies for preventing dental caries. In *Community Oral Health* (C. Pine, ed.). Oxford: Butterworth-Heinemann, pp. 112–125.

Bush, L. A., Horenkamp, N., Morley, J. E. and Spiro, A. (1996). D-E-N-T-A-L: a rapid self-administered screening instrument to promote referrals for further evaluation in older adults. *J. Am. Geriatr. Soc.*, **44**, 478–481.

Carlsson, G. E. (1976). Symptoms of mandibular dysfunction in complete denture wearers. *J. Dent.*, **4**, 265–270.

Carmichael, C. L., Rugg-Gunn, A. J. and Ferrell, R. S. (1989). The relationship between fluoridation, social class and caries experience in 5-year-old children in Newcastle and Northumberland in 1987. *Br. Dent. J.*, **167**, 57–61.

Castle, P. (1987). *The Politics of Water Fluoridation: The Campaign for Fluoridation in the West Midlands of England*. London: John Libbey.

Catford, J. and Nutbeam, D. (1984). Towards a definition of health education and health promotion. *Health Educ. J.*, **43**, 38.

Cheng, L. R. (1990). Asian-American cultural perspectives on birth defects: focus on cleft palate. *Cleft Palate J.*, **27**, 294–300.

Cornwell, J. (1984). *Hard Earned Lives: Accounts of Health and Illness from East London*. London: Tavistock.

Cushing, A., Sheiham, A. and Maizels, J. (1986). Developing socio-dental indicators – the social impact of dental disease. *Community Dent. Health*, **3**, 3–17.

Davey-Smith, G., Bartley, M. and Blane, D. (1990). The Black report on socio-economic inequalities in health 10 years on. *B. M. J.*, **301**, 373–377.

Department of Health (1994). *An Oral Health Strategy for England*. London: DoH.

de Vries, H. C., Lucker, T. P., Cremers, S. B. and Katan, M. B. (1990). Food choice and caries experience in Dutch teenagers as a function of the level of education of their parents. *Eur. J. Clin. Nutr.*, **4**, 839–846.

d'Houtard, A. and Field, M. G. (1984). The image of Health: variations in perceptions by social class in a French population. *Sociology of Health and Illness*, **6**, 30–60.

Douglass, C. W. and Cole, K. (1979). The supply of dental manpower in the United States. *Am. J. Dent. Educ.*, **43**, 287–302.

Downer, M. (1994). Caries prevalence in the United Kingdom. *Int. Dent. J.*, **44**, 367–370.

Downer, M. C. (1995). The 1993 national survey of children's dental health. *Br. Dent. J.*, **178**, 407–412.

Ellwood, R. E. and O'Mullane, D. M. (1995). The association between oral deprivation and dental caries in groups with and without fluoride in their drinking water. *Community Dent. Health*, **12**, 18–22.

Evans, D. J., Rugg-Gunn, A. J., Tabari, E. D. and Butler, T. (1996). The effect of fluoridation and social class on caries experience in 5-year-old Newcastle children in 1994 compared with results over the previous 18 years. *Community Dent. Health*, **13**, 5–10.

Freire, M., de Melo, R. B. and Almeida, S. (1996). Dental caries prevalence in relation to socio-economic status of nursery school children in Goiania-GO, Brazil. *Community Dent. Oral Epidemiol.*, **24**, 357–361.

Haraldson, T., Karlsson, U. and Carlsson, G. (1979). Bite force and oral function in complete denture wearers. *J. Oral Rehabil.*, **6**, 41–48.

Gratrix, D. and Holloway, P. J. (1994). Factors of deprivation associated with dental caries in young children. *Community Dent. Health*, **11**, 66–70.

Herzlich, C. (1973). *Health and Illness*. London: Academic Press.

Heyink, J. W., Heezen, J. and Schaub R. (1986). Dentist and patient appraisal of complete denture in a Dutch elderly poulation. *Community Dent. Oral Epidemiol.*, **14**, 323–326.

Hochstein, J. R., Athanasopoulos, D. and Larkins, J. (1968). Poverty area under the microscope. *Am. J. Public Health*, **58**, 1815–1827.

Holt, R. D., Winter, G. B., Downer, M. C., et al. (1996). Caries in pre-school children in Camden 1993–94. *Br. Dent. J.*, **181**, 405–410.

Hopkins, A. and Bahl, V. (1993). Editors' note. In *Access to Health Care for People from Black and Ethnic Minorities* (A. Hopkins and V. Bahl, eds). London: Royal College of Physicians.

Hopper, S. V. (1993). The influence of ethnicity on the health of older women. *Clin. Geriatr. Med.*, **9**, 231–259.

Howlett, B. C., Ahmad, W. I. and Murray R. (1992). An exploration of White, Asian and Afro-Caribbean peoples' concepts of health and illness causation. *New Comm.*, **18**, 281–292.

Jarman, B. (1984). Identification of underpriveliged areas. *B. M. J.*, **286**, 1705–1709.

Keogh, T. and Linden, G. J. (1991). Knowledge, attitudes and behaviour in relation to dental health of adults in Belfast, Northern Ireland. *Community Dent. Oral Epidemiol.*, **19**, 246–248.

King, J. (1978). Patterns of sugar consumption in early infancy. *Community Dent. Oral Epidemiol.*, **6**, 47–52.

Krasse, B. (1996). The caries decline: is the effect of fluoride toothpaste overrated? *Eur. J. Oral Sci.*, **104**, 426–429.

Kressin, N., Spiro, A., Bosse R., et al. (1996). Assessing oral health-related quality of life: findings from the normative aging study. *Med. Care*, **34**, 416–427.

Laher, M. H. E. (1990). A comparison between dental caries, gingival health and dental service usage in Bangladeshi and white Caucasian children aged 7, 9, 11,

13 and 15 years residing in an inner city area of London, UK. *Community Dent. Health*, **7**, 157–163.

Leao, A. and Sheiham, A. (1995). Relation between clinical dental status and subjective impacts on daily living. *J. Dent. Res.*, **74**, 1408–1413.

Lee, J. (1991). The reorganisation of the City of Toronto dental services: a community development model. *J. Public Health Dent.*, **51**, 99–102.

Lee, K. I., Schwarz, E. and Mak, K. Y. (1993). Improving oral health through understanding the meaning of health and disease in a Chinese culture. *Int. Dent. J.*, **43**, 2–8.

Leeds, D. (1988). *Powerspeak. The Complete Guide to Public Speaking Presentations.* London: Piatkus.

Locker, D. (1988). Measuring oral health: a conceptual framework. *Community Dent. Health*, **9**, 109–124.

Locker, D. and Ford, J. (1994). Evaluation of an area based measure as an indicator of inequalities in oral health. *Community Dent. Oral Epidemiol.*, **22**, 80–85.

Locker, D. and Liddell, A. (1991). Clinical correlates of dental anxiety among older adults. *Community Dent. Oral Epidemiol.*, **20**, 372–375.

Locker, D., Liddell, A. and Burman, D. (1991). Dental fear and anxiety in an older adult population. *Community Dent. Oral Epidemiol.*, **19**, 120–124.

MacEntee, M. I., Hill, P M., Wong, G., Mojon, P., Berkowitz, J. and Glick, N. (1991). Predicting concerns for the mouth among institutionalised elders. *J. Public Health Dent.*, **51**, 82–90.

Magnusson, T. (1980). Prevalence of recurrent headache and mandibular dysfunction in patients with unsatisfactory dentures. *Community Dent. Oral Epidemiol.*, **8**, 159–164.

Mautsch, W. and Sheiham, A. (eds) (1995). *Promoting Oral Health in Deprived Communities.* Berlin: DSE.

McKeown, T. (1979). *The Role of Medicine: Dream, Mirage or Nemesis?* Oxford: Blackwell Scientific.

Milio, N. (1986). *Promoting Health Through Public Policy.* Ottawa: Canadian Public Health Association.

Moynihan, P.J. and Holt, R. D. (1996). The national diet and nutrition survey of 1.5 to 4.5 year old children: summary of the findings of the dental survey. *Br. Dent. J.*, **181**, 328–332.

Murray, J. J. (1994). Comments on results reported at the second international conference 'Changes in caries prevalence'. *Int. Dent. J.*, **44**, 457–458.

Murray, J. J. (1996). Attendance patterns and oral health. *Br. Dent. J.*, **181**, 339–342.

Murray, J. J., Breckon, J. A., Reynolds, P. J., et al. (1991). The effect of residence and social class on dental caries experience in 15–16-year-old children living in three towns (natural fluoride, adjusted fluoride and low fluoride) in the north east of England. *Br. Dent. J.*, **171**, 319–322.

Nadanovsky, P. and Sheiham, A. (1994). The relative contribution of dental services to the changes and geographical variations in caries of 5 and 12 year old children in England and Wales in the 1980s. *Community Dent. Health*, **11**, 215–223.

Nadanovsky, P. and Sheiham, A. (1995). Relative contribution of dental services to the changes in caries levels of 12-year-old children in 18 industrialised countries in the 1970s and early 1980s. *Community Dent. Oral Epidemiol.*, **23**, 331–339.

Normark, S. (1993). Social indicators of dental caries among Sierra Leonean schoolchildren. *Scand. J. Dent. Res.*, **101**, 121–129.

Oakley, A. (1993) *Essays on Women, Medicine and Health.* Edinburgh: Edinburgh University Press.

O'Mullane, D., Whelton, H. and Galvin, N. (1993). Health services and women's oral health. *J. Dent. Educ.*, **57**, 749–752.

OPCS (1980). *Classification of Occupations*. London: HMSO.

Peter, J. and Chinsky, R. (1974). Sociological aspects of cleft palate adults I: marriage. *Cleft Palate J.*, **11**, 259–309.

Petersson, G. H. and Bratthall, D. (1996). The caries decline: a review of reviews. *Eur. J. Oral Sci.*, **104**, 436–443.

Petridou, E., Athanassouli, T., Panagopoulos, H. and Revinthi, K. (1996). Sociodemographic and dietary factors in relation to dental health among Greek adolescents. *Community Dent. Oral Epidemiol,.* **24**, 307–311.

Pill, R. and Stott, N. C. H. (1982). Concepts of illness causation and responsibility: some preliminary data from a sample of working class mothers. *Soc. Sci. Med.*, **16**, 43–52.

Prendergast, M. J., Beal, J. F. and Williams, S. A. (1997). The relationship between deprivation, ethnicity and dental health in 5-year-old children in Leeds, UK. *Community Dent. Health*, **14**, 18–21.

Reisine, S. T. (1988). The effects of pain and oral health on the quality of life. Community Dent. Health, **5**, 63–68.

Sarll, D. W., Whittle, J. G. and Mackie, I. C. (1984). The use of a classification of residential registration (ACORN) as a health-related variable in service planning for dentistry. *Community Dent. Health*, **1**, 115–123.

Sakki, T. K., Knuuttila, M. L., Vimpari, S. S., et al. (1994). Lifestyle, dental caries and number of teeth. *Community Dent. Oral Epidemiol.*, **22**, 298–302.

Schou, L. and Uitenbroek, D. (1995). Social and behavioural indicators of caries experience in 5-year-old children. *Community Dent. Oral Epidemiol.*, **23**, 276–281.

Shaw, W. C., Rees, G., Dawe, M. and Charles, C. R. (1985). The influence of dentofacial appearance on the social attractiveness of young adults. *Am. J. Orthod.*, **87**, 21–26.

Silver, D. H. (1992). A comparison of 3-year-olds' caries experience in 1973, 1981 and 1989 in a Hertfordshire town, related to family behaviour and social class. *Br. Dent. J.*, **172**, 191–197.

Slade, G. D. and Spencer, A. J. (1994). Development and evaluation of the Oral Health Impact Profile. *Community Dent. Health*, **11**, 3–11.

Slade, G. D., Spencer, A. J., Davies, M. J. and Stewart, J. F. (1996). The influence of exposure to fluoridated water on socio-economic inequalities in children's caries experience. *Community Dent. Oral Epidemiol.*, **24**, 89–100.

Smith, J. P. (1977). Observer variation in the clinical diagnosis of mandibular pain dysfunction syndrome. *Community Dent. Oral Epidemiol.*, **8**, 360–364.

Smith, J. and Sheiham, A. (1979). How dental conditions handicap the elderly. *Community Dent. Oral Epidemiol.*, **7**, 305–310.

Soh, G. (1992). Racial differences in perception of oral health and oral health behaviours in Singapore. *Int. Dent. J.*, **42**, 234–240.

Steele, J. G., Walls, A. W., Ayatollahi, S. M., et al. (1996). Major clinical findings from a dental survey of elderly people in three different English communities. *Br. Dent. J.*, **180**, 17–23.

Thomas, J. F. and Startup, R. (1992). Some social correlates with the dental health of young children. *Community Dent. Health*, **9**, 11–17.

Thomson, W. M. and Cautley, A. J. (1996). Self-reported dental status and treatment need among elderly people. *N. Z. Dent. J.*, **92**, 105–109.

Thomson, W. M., Spencer, A. J. and Gaughwin, A. (1996). Testing a child dental neglect scale in South Australia. *Community Dent. Oral Epidemiol.*, **24**, 351–356.

Todd, J. and Lader, D. (1991). *Adult Dental Health, 1988, UK*. London: HMSO.

Whittle, J. G. and Davies, K. W. (1992). A classification of residential neighbourhoods (ACORN) in relation to dental health and dental health behaviours. *Community Dent. Health*, **9**, 217–224.

Williams, R. (1983). Concepts of health: an analysis of lay logic. *Sociology*, **17**, 185–204.

Williams, S. A. (1984). Infant feeding practices and dental health. *Community Dent. Health*, **1**, 78 (abstract).

Williams, S. A. and Fairpo, C. (1988). Cultural variations in oral hygiene practices among infants resident in an inner city area. *Community Dent. Health*, **5**, 265–271.

World Health Organization (1948). *Constitution*. Geneva: WHO.

World Health Organization (1980). *International Classification of Impairments, Disabilities and Handicaps*. Geneva: WHO.

World Health Organization (1984). *Health Promotion. A Discussion Document on the Concept and Principles*. Copenhagen: Regional Office for Europe.

World Health Organization (1995). *Oral Health Programme. 12 Year Book/95.3*. Geneva: WHO.

Uba, L. (1992). Cultural barriers to health care for southeastern Asian refugees. *Public Health Rep.*, **107**, 544–548.

Chapter 3

Lay and professional contributions to oral health

In this chapter, the ideas outlined in the previous chapter are developed, focusing upon the range of dental activity that is carried out both outside and within the dental surgery. We begin with an important distinction between formal and informal oral health care and use some implications of the previous chapter to explain why only a minority of people use formal dental services. We build upon the possible range of ideas that different people may have about health and consider the importance of these ideas in the context of accessing formally organized dental care. Alternative ideas about understanding the relationship between professionals and lay people are then reviewed. The process of becoming a dentist is described and the personal outcomes of this are assessed.

Formal and informal oral health care activity

Stacey (1993) clarified what activities should be included when people attempt to maintain their health: what she termed 'health work'. She proposed that there is an important distinction between what health professionals accomplish in their work and what lay people accomplish in their everyday lives. Health care professionals, including all members of the primary dental care team, have undergone specialist training and are paid for their work. They provide the formal aspects of health work.

However, Stacey pointed out that a great many more people also contribute to the maintenance of health and the provision of care during illness. There are many more informal than formal health workers. Because in many cultures women take on much of the responsibility for health in families, most of this informal health care work will be supplied by women. The production of good health begins with childbirth and continues with the socialization of children, and it can involve many aspects of self-care, including caring for our own bodies, family care, self-help groups in the community and community care. The distinction between formal and informal health work is of most value in industrialized societies where there is a complex division of labour, for example, where there are primary dental care team members who each have specific skills and responsibilities.

The use of this distinction in dental care

Formal care services rely on informal care-givers to ensure good health. For example, dentists rely on parents to restrict their children's diet and to teach them the importance of oral hygiene during the socialization process. If lay members of society did not form their own care networks, the dental profession would be overwhelmed by disease. The importance of this is illustrated by the attempts to encourage self-care, as shown by the publication of self-care advice to the public on the prevention of dental disease (Health Education Authority, 1996). This advice is summarized as:

- Reduce the consumption and especially the frequency of intake of sugar-containing food and drink.
- Clean the teeth thoroughly twice every day with a fluoride toothpaste.
- Request the local water supply company to adjust to the optimum fluoride content.
- Have an oral examination by a dentist every year.

These are explicit attempts to encourage the informal health care system. The emphasis is upon individuals developing control over aspects of their diet and oral hygiene. There is evidence that populations are improving their oral hygiene activity, with most people in industrialized countries brushing their teeth one to two times a day (Sheiham and Croucher, 1994). As people develop these informal health care skills, their understanding and practice of what is appropriate behaviour in terms of diet and oral hygiene may affect their relationship with formal health care workers (Gerhardt, 1989). There could be both positive and negative effects of this increased sense of control. If people feel confident about their personal knowledge and skills, then they might develop a greater sense of competence. However, at the same time, they might not readily accept the value of what a dentist says. On the one hand, the informal health workers are expected to accept responsibility for personal health and know when they should access the formal care system, but on the other hand they are expected to be passive when meeting the professional. This has been described as a 'double bind'.

In general, studies of the dentist–patient relationship have not considered this double bind in detail. Research has been mainly concerned with variations in the behaviour, feelings and attitudes of patients as these relate to patient management (Linn, 1971; Ayer and Corah, 1984). Locker (1989) has also noted that there has been a tendency to see dentistry merely as a set of procedures performed on patients. Patients' views are not taken seriously. There is little recognition of the significance of the formal/informal health activity distinction and the implications that this might have for understanding the professional–lay person consultation.

Implicit in this also is the lack of recognition of lay ideas about health that may be brought to the consultation. In practical terms, it is known that a better quality of interaction leads to more reported satisfaction with health care which, in turn, leads to positive health outcomes. These issues are demonstrated by the work of Arnbjerg et al. (1992) who investigated the satisfaction with previous dental care of a Swedish population aged 45–69 years. Satisfaction with previous dental care depended primarily on three factors: treatment by the dentist of choice; chewing ability; and contentment with their own dental conditions.

The clinical iceberg

One outcome of the finding that informal health workers may have particular ideas about the management of symptoms is the discovery in many surveys of what has been termed the 'clinical iceberg'. When people are asked to keep diaries of their health symptoms, many more symptoms are recorded in the diaries than are actually reported to the formal health care system (Wadsworth et al., 1971). Thus, health professionals see only a small part of the illness in the community, just as only a small part of an iceberg is visible above the surface of the water. There is a large discrepancy between the need for medical and dental care and the demand for formal health care services. Self-care is used to treat many symptoms. A gradient of the likelihood of symptom experience leading to a consultation has also been established (Banks et al., 1975). People are much more likely to consult if they have a major disabling or threatening symptom, such as pain in the chest, than if they feel the symptom is more minor, such as a change in energy.

There are many oral health examples of this phenomenon. The UK national surveys of adult dental health, conducted every 10 years, usually report an almost universal presence of the clinical signs of gingivitis and periodontal disease in the general population. Similarly, Locker (1989) asked a sample of Canadians to report any symptoms of oral or facial pain in the previous four weeks. Forty per cent reported at least one symptom within this time period, but of these only 44% had sought professional attention. Indeed, only 62%

of those with severe toothache had sought formal help. This finding was not dissimilar to those reported by Anderson and Newman (1973), who found that 75% of their respondents with toothache would visit the dentist, 61% with tooth loss, 54% with sensitivity to hot or cold and 45% with sore or bleeding gums. As with general health, there is a gradient of response to symptoms.

One problem with these kind of surveys is that they rely on respondents' self-reports of their health and behaviour. There is some evidence that this information needs to be treated with considerable caution, even though in many situations self-report can provide the only source of readily available data. A common question asked in surveys concerns the regularity of dental attendance. One study found that for dentate adults, 48% claimed that they attended for regular check-ups, 13% that they attended for the occasional check-up, and 40% only when they were experiencing some trouble with their teeth. Eddie (1984) put such claims to the test by consulting a sample population's dental records. Of those who claimed regular attendance, only 31% had actually done so in the previous five years, 53% had attended infrequently, and 16% not at all. Perhaps the respondents in surveys are replying according to their beliefs about how they should behave, rather than on the basis of their actual behaviour.

A second problem focuses on the definition of need that is used in the surveys. Usually professionally defined (normative) need is used, which may have little relationship with lay (felt or expressed) need (Bradshaw, 1972). A difference between the two often exists. A professional definition of need usually relies on the presence of disease, which is a more exclusive definition than the lay ideas of health that were described in the previous chapter. In the next section of this chapter, we consider some of the factors that influence whether a person will seek professional help for symptoms.

Health behaviour and illness behaviour

A useful distinction that summarizes the issues raised in this chapter can be gained from the terms 'health behaviour' and 'illness behaviour'. Originally defined by Kasl and Cobb (1966), *health behaviour* has come to mean any activity undertaken by individuals for the purpose of preventing disease or detecting it at an asymptomatic stage. Activities could include flossing the teeth, evaluating diet or attending for a dental check-up. *Illness behaviour* is any activity undertaken by individuals who perceive themselves as having a health problem for the purpose of defining their health and discovering and undertaking an appropriate remedy. Both definitions imply that there is not automatic use of the formal health care system.

Many models have been proposed to explain illness behaviour, but they have the common features of:

- Accessibility to health care.
- Evaluation of that health care.
- Perceptions of the symptoms.
- Social network characteristics, i.e. the number and quality of the relationships that an individual has with other informal health workers who can be consulted about the perceived health problem.
- Knowledge about the disease.
- Demographic characteristics, such as age, sex and social class.

Factors affecting the decision to consult

As noted earlier, there is a considerable symptom iceberg in the community, meaning that many illness episodes are accepted by people without seeking a professional intervention. Three separate sets of ideas have been proposed as influencing the decision to consult a professional.

Triggers to consult

The first of these was outlined by Zola (1973). He noted that many people in doctors' consulting rooms had been suffering from pain and other symptoms for quite considerable lengths of time before consulting a professional. Often, symptoms were tolerated or not seen as sufficient to merit professional care until some event ('the trigger') occurred. Five types of triggers were proposed:

1. **The occurrence of an interpersonal crisis.** There might be a change in personal relationships, such as a domestic crisis, which can change the evaluation of what may have been perceived as an otherwise minor symptom.
2. **Perceived interference with social or personal relations.** Symptoms that interfere with normal social relations may create more concern, such as toothache preventing someone from following recreational activity such as sailing or going on holiday.
3. **Perceived interference with vocational or physical activity.** Symptoms that interfere with the normal activities of daily life will be evaluated as abnormal (see the discussion of impacts in Chapter 2).

4. **Temporalizing of symptomatology.** This involves the potential patient setting a deadline by deciding that they will consult if the symptom has not disappeared by a certain date.
5. **Sanctioning.** This relates to pressure from friends or relatives to use health services.

Lay referral network

This latter process of consultation with friends has been described by Friedson (1970) as accessing the 'lay referral network'. Friedson argued that seeking help involves consulting a network of informal consultants before seeking formal help from a health professional. Often the passage to formal health care may depend upon the degree of similarity of beliefs between informal and formal health carers and the number of informal consultants available. If a person has few friends or relatives to consult and there is consensus of advice from them that a symptom requires attention, then a professional will be consulted sooner. If, however, there is a large number of informal consultants and there is little similarity of beliefs, then the lowest rate of utilization of formal health care will follow.

Lim et al. (1984) investigated the influence of networks of family and friends upon the response of participants in a plaque control programme. The participants were 41 patients who had been referred to a dental hospital for treatment. There was a major reduction in plaque and gingivitis levels in all patients at both the 10th and 14th weeks of the study. However, there was a greater proportional reduction in gingivitis levels in those who reported a higher number of discussions with their friends. The effect of discussions with members of the family was less clear. Lower values for gingivitis levels at 10 weeks were associated with a higher number of discussions with parents, but levels of gingivitis seemed to be adversely affected by discussions between the participants and their spouses. Lim et al. concluded that it was important to recognize the influence of networks when preventive programmes are designed, especially if these involve high levels of self-care.

Meetings between experts

Tuckett et al. (1985) proposed that the lay–professional encounter should be described as 'a meeting between experts'. They argue that this is a useful way of understanding consulting behaviour because these days the professional is no longer perceived as fully knowledgeable and the lay person completely ignorant. Both have their values, expectations and understandings, which may vary. Recognizing this issue will have positive outcomes. The lay person will be more satisfied with the consultation if his or her opinions and skills are recognized. The professional may well have less stress if he or she appreciates the limitations of surgery-based clinical expertise and develops improved communication skills with patients; these issues are explored in greater depth in the following chapters.

Accessing primary dental care

Once a person has made the decision to consult a dentist, there is still the issue of access. Primary dental care – the formal aspect of oral health – is the care provided at the first point of contact. It is necessary to have information about the use of services for planning purposes, both financial and manpower. Increasingly in recent years, patients are being perceived as consumers who can make choices about what services to use and when they might choose to use them.

Penchansky and Thomas (1981) proposed that access was made up of five different facets. These were:

- **Availability:** the relationship between the volume and type of services with the consumers' volume and type of need. Are there enough providers of care and sufficient facilities for them to work in?
- **Accessibility:** the relationship between the location of the supply of services and the location of the consumer, considering issues such as transportation, distance and cost of travel.
- **Accommodation:** the relationship between the organization of the services in terms of opening hours and other services, and the clients' ability to relate to these factors.
- **Affordability:** the relationship of the cost of services to the consumers' ability to pay these costs.
- **Acceptability:** the mutual perceptions that both providers and consumers have of each other, in terms of attributes such as age, sex or ethnicity.

These facets can interlink and have a synergistic effect. The major policy focus has tended to be on the facet of availability. However, as availability decreases, it becomes harder for the consumers to access services. There is a range of evidence identifying what factors are important in explaining the use of services, which have been summarized as epidemiological, demographic, socioeconomic, personal and psychological, and the characteristics of the system (Bauer and Pierson, 1978; see also Anderson and Morgan, 1992, for a review).

The issue of equitable access has also been highlighted. Tudor-Hart

(1971) proposed the 'inverse care law'. This stated that the provision of health care is inversely related to the need for it. This was demonstrated in a study of access to dental services by O'Mullane and Robinson (1984), who investigated the uptake of treatment by 508 14-year-old children in different social classes in two towns in England with different dentist:population ratios. In the town with an unfavourable dentist:population ratio, the uptake of treatment was considerably higher in the higher social classes. In the town with a favourable dentist:population ratio, the uptake was similar throughout the social scale. This suggests that patients from lower social classes are put at a further disadvantage when there are fewer dentists available.

Barriers to care

There are a number of barriers to accessing professional care, including fear and anxiety (see Chapter 4), the cost of treatment and aspects of the dental practice environment. The impact of these different barriers has been evaluated by Todd and Lader (1991). They invited 3500 adults to consider 15 statements: five on aspects of fear, five on the cost of treatment and five on aspects of dental practice organization. A minority of the sample (11%) indicated that they perceived no barriers to dental care, 45% selected a barrier related to fear, and equal numbers (22%) selected barriers related either to practice organization or to cost. Women were more likely to identify with the statements, especially those related to fear, while those respondents who attended only with dental problems were more likely to associate themselves with all the statements, with fear being the most important.

Although self-reports of barriers are informative, some validation of such findings is also needed. While respondents may perceive barriers, it does not necessarily mean that this will have an impact upon their oral health. However, the oral cavity is particularly accessible to examination compared with other parts of the body, and a strength of the Todd and Lader study was that they included a clinical examination of respondents. There were, indeed, correlations between reported barriers due to fear and dental condition. Fearful patients were more likely to have more missing teeth and fewer filled teeth than those not reporting any barrier statements. That these two factors are correlated together does not necessarily propose a causal relationship, which would require further study. However, one practical implication of this finding would appear to be that these patients were delaying accessing treatment until it was difficult for the dentist to provide an adequate restoration.

Patients' perceptions of the dentist

Once individuals decide to access dental care, there can be a feeling of self-controlled resignation about the process of treatment, as these adults commented:

> It's normally a rush, you're in there and out fairly quickly, and most of the time I've got my mouth open with him working in it
> . . .
> I think it's a case of you get in there, let him do what he's got to do, and go ... get it all over and done with ...

These patients apparently adopted similar attitudes to their dentists. The dentist was perceived as knowing what treatment was needed and the patient's role was seen as being cooperative in achieving this. However, feelings about receiving treatment can provoke startling comparisons with other situations, as a third quotation suggests:

> Having had three pregnancies, you kind of get messed around a lot then ... its a similar experience, lying flat on your back, people doing things to you can't really do much about ... (Croucher, 1989, p. 25)

These qualitative findings have been repeated in other quantitative surveys involving large samples of respondents. DiMatteo et al. (1995) investigated public attitudes to dentists using telephone interviewing. They reported that, in their sample of 647 adults, those who were older and with a higher income were more likely to report a greater trust and respect for the dentist. Women also reported this, especially if the dentist was perceived as being sensitive to patient pain or anxiety. The younger respondents and those with a lower income attached greater importance to positive communication and effective diagnosis and treatment. Gerbert et al. (1994) also explored the image of the dentist by sending questionnaires to both dentists and their patients. They concluded that patients are happy with their dentists – an unsurprising finding given that the investigators apparently had little control over which patients were asked to complete the questionnaires by their dentists! There is some evidence that patients and dentists 'shop' for each other until they find one who meets their personal preferences.

As noted earlier, there is always the possibility of conflict in the lay–professional consultation. This is demonstrated in the UK by evidence of patient use of the formal National Health Service complaints procedure against their dentists. Mellor and Milgrom (1995a) investigated this issue using a postal questionnaire. The aim was to establish the prevalence of complaints between 1989 and 1993. Two hundred and eighty-nine dentists responded, of whom 35 per cent had reported at least one potential complaint. Of these, 11 per cent reported that the potential complaint had become an official complaint. Those reporting official complaints were also likely to report a higher number of unsatisfactory patient visits. This finding was developed in a further report (Mellor and Milgrom, 1995b). Dentists who had greater scores relating to unpleasant feelings (e.g. 'I felt depressed after seeing the patient'), lack of communication (e.g. 'we just didn't hit it off') and practice organization (e.g. 'problems in my practice interfered with the visit') were more likely to report official malpractice complaints.

Patients also have clear ideas about the quality of dental care. For 1328 Dutch respondents, the hygiene of instruments and the availability of the dentist in an emergency were considered the most important. This group of respondents – all regular dentist attenders with only a small percentage with low levels of education – placed greater importance upon the technical and functional aspects of care, rather than communication (Goedhart et al., 1996).

Negative perceptions
Perceptions of the dentist may be especially important for special needs groups such as those with HIV. Dentists in the UK are advised to provide care for patients with HIV but not with AIDS, in the context of a universal level of infection control. There is no clinical reason for these patients not to be treated by their general dental practitioner. However, Robinson et al. (1994) established from their study of 146 men with HIV that half of those who had been to the dentist since being given their HIV diagnosis had withheld this information in order to secure treatment. Of those who revealed their diagnosis to the dentist, half had been either refused treatment or offered only limited treatment. Commonly voiced concerns were related to the attitudes of the members of the dental team and concerns about confidentiality.

Negative perceptions of the dentist were also reported by a sample of irregular attenders (Finch et al., 1988). Dentists were associated with pain, being impersonal and being highly paid. As these were irregular attenders, it may be argued that these perceptions reflect a set of expectations based around early experience, which may have little basis in the current reality of dental practice. One respondent summarized her perception of the dentist by reporting that 'they see you as a mouth'.

With the increasing recognition that patients' perceptions of their dentists are significant not only for their satisfaction but also for their willingness to access formal treatment, Smith et al. (1984) developed the Dental Beliefs Survey (DBS). The DBS consists of 28 statements, and patients indicate their degree of agreement or disagreement with each one. Some of the statements concern professionalism and ethics (e.g. 'When a dentist seems in a hurry I worry that I'm not getting good care' and 'Dentists focus too much on getting the work done and not enough on the patient's comfort'); other statements are about communication (e.g. 'I feel dentists do not provide clear explanations' and 'I am concerned that dentists do not like to take the time to really talk to patients'), and others are about lack of control (e.g. 'I am concerned that the dentist will do what he wants and not really listen to me while I'm in the chair').

Is there an ideal dentist and patient?

From the studies reported in the previous section, it is apparent that the findings depend to a large extent on who is surveyed. Van Groenistijn et al. (1980) asked 513 randomly selected Dutch adults about the features of an ideal dentist. Whilst there was general agreement about the key features of the ideal dentist, these varied according to the social class of the respondent. The commonly agreed positive features were professional skill, ability to put the patient at ease and friendliness. Respondents of higher social class placed greater emphasis upon professional skill and explanation of treatment, whilst the respondents of lower social class emphasized reassurance and friendliness. This work was developed by Lahti et al. (1996), who reviewed previous studies to develop a questionnaire which was administered to 50 dentists and 100 patients in Finland. Both groups of respondents agreed that one characteristic of the ideal dentist was the importance of mutual communication, whilst a common feature of the ideal patient was manageability.

Collett (1969) also asked dentists about their ideal patient, who was seen to be aged between 25 and 55 years, female, well-educated and from the upper social classes. This study also reported that half of the dentists responding had lost patients due to poor interpersonal relations.

Models of the lay–professional relationship

Such results illustrate the importance of considering the nature of the relationship between dentist and patient. This section will consider two major attempts to develop models of the lay–professional relationship. The first of these was the work of Parsons (1951), who coined the term 'the sick role', whilst the second was developed by Szasz and Hollender (1956).

The sick role

Parsons (1951) proposed that when people are ill they enter the sick role, which allows them both privileges and obligations. If a patient accepts the sick role, he or she ought to:

- Want to get well as quickly as possible.
- Seek professional advice and cooperate with that advice.
- Be allowed to shed some normal activities and responsibilities, such as domestic and paid employment.

In return, the health professional is expected to apply a high degree of skill and knowledge, act for the welfare of the patient and the community rather than out of self-interest, be emotionally detached and be guided by the rules of professional practice. In return for these expectations, health professionals are granted the right to conduct physical examinations, have an autonomous professional practice and act in a position of authority in relation to patients.

However, Parsons' ideas have been criticized on several grounds. Parsons proposes a passive patient, who is regarded as being in need of care and unable to get better by him- or herself. The model accepts inequality between patient and professional with equanimity and does not recognize the ideas of informal care and lay competence proposed in this chapter. Although it might be appropriate for an acute disease situation (as when a person is seriously ill), it does not apply particularly well to chronic diseases, which are the most common type of illness in modern industrialized societies.

Gerson (1972) investigated whether the idea of the sick role could be applied to dental as well as to medical problems. By asking members of the general population about their views, he established that similar sick role exemptions are expected for dental as well as medical problems. However, the amount of expected exemption is greater for medical than for dental problems. His respondents did not feel that they could stay away from their normal activities and responsibilities for as long with a dental condition as they could for a medical one.

This finding has had a recent practical application. Traditionally, oral surgery can involve a formal two- or three-day inpatient admission. In a study by Greenwood (1993), 200 patients were asked for their views of day case oral surgery. The most commonly reported advantage of this procedure was reported as less disruption to normal routine. Respondents did not feel bound to accept the sick role. Interestingly, however, a small minority were concerned that being asked to recover at home would not allow them adequate rest. Their right to adopt the privileges of the sick role would be limited.

The Szasz and Hollender model

This second approach to the lay–professional relationship also involves ideas of responsibility and authority, but in a different way. Instead of trying to describe an ideal, Szasz and Hollender (1956) observed that there are three types of relationship:

- **Active–passive.** Here the health professional assumes complete responsibility for the patient, who is in a state of collapse or under a general anaesthetic.
- **Guidance–cooperation.** The health professional instructs the patient on what needs to be done about the complaint, and the patient follows this advice.
- **Mutual participation.** This is a cooperative relationship where each shares responsibility. In this situation, the patient accepts day-to-day responsibility for the management of his or her symptoms while the health professional provides input when needed.

A possible fourth type can also be proposed: the *passive–active* relationship. This might be the situation where the patient becomes a consumer and directs the practitioner to provide certain services. This might be the case in certain types of cosmetic dentistry or where there is an oversupply of dentists.

Both Parsons and Szasz and Hollender assume that there is underlying consensus within the lay–professional relationship. However, Friedson (1970) suggested that there is potential for conflict between the separate worlds of informal and formal health care. A dentist might be working with one model, for example, expecting a patient to take on the sick role and follow advice without argument, while the patient may have a very different view. In such an instance there could be the need for improved communication.

Dentist–patient communication

Szasz and Hollender proposed that the mutual participation model should be adopted as the most preferable in the context of chronic disease and preventive care. Its basis in cooperation and communication might also allow the opportunity for the ideas and competencies of informal health care workers to be placed alongside those of formal health care workers. However, there is little evidence that this occurs in practice. Wanless and Holloway (1994) analysed the audio-recordings of a group of 30 general dental practitioners with 132 patients aged 10–17 years. Whilst consultations were found to have a consistent structure composed of a sequence of stages overall, not all of these stages were present in each consultation. Basic features were not observed by some dentists, such as greeting the patient and using the patient's name. Patients who asked questions were not always given a reply, and in only 19% of cases was the purpose of the visit explained. Where advice on tooth brushing was provided, it was very rare for good methods to be actually demonstrated.

This has been described by Croucher (1989) as 'the performance gap'. In his study of 150 adult patients who were receiving preventive treatment for gum disease in general dental practice, many were found to be confused as to why they were receiving their treatment. The patients did not get the advice they were expecting on a wide range of issues. Explanations for the advice they were offered was often not forthcoming. Croucher proposed that there was a need for dentists to establish the information needs of each patient.

Becoming a dentist

These results reinforce the point made in Chapter 1 that the professional preparation of dentists should include a wider range of skills, including communication skills. Communication skills are considered in more detail in Chapter 9, but here we examine some of the research on the process of becoming a formal oral health care worker such as a dentist.

Socialization into dentistry

The concept of primary socialization has already been highlighted in Chapter 2 as an important way of recognizing the way that lay self-care health behaviours are developed in childhood. This concept can also be applied to becoming a dentist. In this case it is *secondary socialization* that should be considered. This is mainly transmitted in Western societies through educational and work institutions, whilst training in dental school involves a specific process of professional socialization. This involves learning not only many technical skills but also how to behave like a professional.

The bulk of a student's undergraduate and postgraduate socialization into dentistry involves the acquisition of specialist knowledge and technical skills, but this is only part of the process. Students also learn about the ways that dentists are expected to behave and dress in front of patients. They are expected to gain an appropriate professional attitude towards their work. Some aspects of socialization are informal, as when a teacher mentions that a white coat is not as clean as it could be, or when students watch interactions between staff members and patients. Other socialization pressures are formal, as when students learn about the legislation passed by governments or the role of professional organizations.

Research on the effects of professional socialization can be performed either by following the same group of students through their course (called a longitudinal design) or by looking at different groups of students from different years (called a cross-sectional design). Shuval (1975) has suggested that there are similar basic professional orientations of students during the first three years of professional socialization in four health fields in Israel. In this longitudinal study, data were analysed from groups of medical, dental, pharmacy and nursing students at three points: prior to entry to the course; at the end of the first year; and at the end of the third year. It seems that professional socialization is a uniform process across different areas of health.

In a study of the professional socialization of dental hygienists, an attempt was made to identify and assess the degree of influence that different role models in education and practice had on the professional socialization of dental hygiene graduates. Two themes were investigated within professional socialization: attitudes toward professionalism and interpersonal values. Dental hygiene graduates were asked to indicate whether they did or did not identify with a dental hygiene role model based around either school or work. Those respondents who identified with a role model based around school had significantly stronger positive attitudes towards their professional organization. Those dental hygienists who identified with a work-based role model had stronger positive interpersonal values. Those graduates who did not identify with either a school- or work-based role model placed greater emphasis on feeling independent (Kraemer, 1990).

These findings emphasize that socialization – in childhood or in later life – is not necessarily a uniform process and that, depending upon who and what are considered important by the student, different outcomes may result.

Stress

Dentistry has a reputation for being a particularly stressful occupation. Indeed, Cooper et al. (1988) indicated that dentistry can be extremely stressful, with ratings being one of the highest of all professions. However, it is possible to overemphasize the difficulties faced by dentists. Comparisons between dentists and other health professionals indicate that they do not have an appreciably higher prevalence of physical morbidity: other professionals have physical and psychological problems too. A high rate of suicide is a widely quoted statistic, but in fact the research on this is based on extremely small numbers and cannot be considered reliable (Kent, 1987). Some studies have shown a lower rate than expected for age and race (Dean, 1969; Hill and Harvey, 1972).

Stress in dental school

The stresses reported by students depend to some extent on their year of the course, but academic concerns relating to the volume of material (rather than with conceptual difficulty) are generally rated highly. Inconsistent feedback from staff is often a problem (Goldstein, 1979). Sachs et al. (1981) identified several concerns. These included relationships with teachers (e.g. 'being treated as though you were immature and irresponsible' and 'dealing with authoritarian, unsympathetic instructors'), academic worries (e.g. 'being unable to learn everything' and 'fear of making a mistake'), feeling lonely, and financial troubles.

Recognition that such problems are widespread among dentists and dental students can itself be reassuring. It is 'normal' for students to be anxious when initially treating patients, or for experienced dentists to be concerned about the possibility of a medical emergency (Cooper et al., 1987). It is common for health professionals to believe that they should be able to cope with their professional lives with little difficulty and to feel ashamed if they cannot. This belief often inhibits individuals from discussing their problems with others. The relief experienced when someone discovers that his or her difficulties are being experienced by colleagues can be profound.

Stress in dental practice

When Godwin et al. (1981) asked recent graduates to describe 'the sources of greatest stress', 73% mentioned patient management (which included some reference to patient fear and anxiety, late or missed appointments and patient dissatisfaction with their services), 50% reported business management problems (such as collection of fees, cash flow problems, overheads and insurance), and 38% mentioned the frustrations due to the discrepancy between their treatment expectations generated within the dental school and the realities of day-to-day dentistry. Problems with patients may arise partly from a lack of awareness of the contribution that a patient can make to a successful consultation.

In Godwin et al.'s study, 26% of graduates indicated that time pressure, particularly when they fell behind schedule, was a source of stress. Problems with staff management were also cited by 33%. The acquisition of effective management skills (Emling, 1980) is important here, especially since Locker et al. (1989) found that one of the main sources of dental assistants' stress was feeling undervalued by the dentist. A more recent study (Newton and Gibbons, 1996) has indicated similar results.

There is also some work on the incidence of major problems, such as the death of a patient under general anaesthetic or other serious reactions to drugs. In Young's (1975) survey, 43% of the dentists involved had experienced at least one occasion within the previous five years when resuscitation was necessary. While the incidence for specific problems was low (e.g. for respiratory arrest it was 0.02 cases per dentist per year), the average practitioner may worry about his or her ability to respond appropriately should an emergency occur. Such a concern was illustrated by one dentist who claimed that he had given a large number of general anaesthetics over the past 10 years without trouble, but added the rider 'so something has to happen soon'.

The type of practice that a dentist has may also be important. Russek (1962) posted questionnaires to dentists in four specialties that were considered to involve varying levels of stress: general practice (most); oral surgery; orthodontics; and periodontology (least). After the results were adjusted for age, there was a gradation in the number of heart complaints reported by the dentists. Those in general practice reported almost three times the incidence of coronary heart disease than those in periodontology. Whether these differences were due solely to the relative stressfulness of the specialities or partly influenced by self-selection into the specialities cannot be ascertained from this study. It may be that the kinds of dentists who choose general practice or oral surgery are more prone to heart disease than those who choose orthodontics or period-ontology.

Not only dentists experience stress, and there is an increasing amount of research on the difficulties faced by other members of the dental team, such as dental assistants. Surveys in both Europe and North America have provided similar results, with assistants indicating that there are a number of commonly encountered sources of stress. These complement those reported by dentists to some degree and include running behind time, feeling undervalued by the dentist, lack of recognition, low income and handling difficult patients (Craven et al., 1995). These stresses are associated not only with intentions to change job, but also with lowered emotional well-being and job satisfaction (Locker, 1996).

Models and measures of stress

One of the more popular approaches to the understanding of occupational stress is provided by the Demand–Control, or job strain, model of stress. According to this model, poor health and subjective feelings of stress are due to the joint effect of a perceived high level of demand coupled with a perceived low level of control over these demands. Such demands could include having to work fast, having to work hard, having a great deal of work to do and not having enough time to do it. Although such demands can have negative effects in themselves, the model also postulates that their effects can be exacerbated when an individual believes that he or she has little control over them. If there is little authority and opportunity to make decisions (and have them implemented) or to control the speed at which work is done, then demands can become significant sources of stress (Baker et al., 1996).

One idea that has been used to describe the effects of stress is known as burnout. Maslach (1982) described three aspects of burnout: emotional exhaustion (or EE), which refers to a sense of being emotionally drained by the work; depersonalization (or DP), which refers to a sense of alienation where patients begin to be treated as impersonal objects rather than valued recipients of care; and personal accomplishment (PA), which refers to the sense of accomplishment that we all need to feel, i.e. that our work is valued and valuable. As a person becomes more stressed by his or her job, EE and DP increase, while the sense of PA lessens.

A person's level of burnout can be measured by the Maslach Burnout Inventory, which consists of a series of 22 statements designed to measure each of the three aspects. When Osborne and Croucher (1994) sent this questionnaire to a group of dentists, high levels of burnout symptoms were found among those who replied. Approximately 11% of the dentists could be said to be suffering from burnout, indicating a significant and serious problem within the profession.

Stress management

The training in communication skills mentioned in Chapter 9 can help to reduce stress. Not only does such training benefit the dentist–patient relationship, but it also increases confidence and the ability to handle difficult situations. The same principles apply to relationships with staff as well. However, there are several other more direct ways to reduce stress. O'Shea et al. (1984) found that practising dentists used a variety of strategies, including exercise, taking time off work, and hobbies. Although such methods are effective in the short run, they involve avoiding rather than attempting to change the situation. The programme advocated by Bosmajian and Bosmajian (1983) provides a structured approach to change. They argue that stress can only be reduced if an individual is first aware of those situations which cause stress. To this end, they provide a 'stresslog'. Dentists are encouraged to note the situations where stress occurs, what the events imply, and what responses were made. The completion of such a diary allows a dentist to see repeating patterns in both events and responses. Once a detailed record is made over several weeks, a pattern may emerge. The stresslog may indicate that a dentist is frequently frustrated by the quality of his or her work due to time pressures, and this could be related to some of the erroneous assumptions that dentists often make about their practice, such as those suggested by Ireland (1983):

1. I should be appreciated by every patient.
2. To be worthwhile, I must be thoroughly competent and successful in my field.
3. I should be emotionally concerned for every patient.
4. There is always a right, precise and perfect solution to a patient's problems, and this solution must always be found.

Having such high and unrealistic expectations about one's own performance will almost certainly result in stress when these standards cannot be met.

Alternatively, a dentist may find that the most stressful situations involve relationships with other members of the dental team. Students may identify a completely different set of stresses. For some it could be a lack of confidence in dealing with patients, while for others it could be anxiety about the workload. Stress management programmes have been evaluated and shown to be effective (Tisdelle et al., 1984).

Summary

This chapter has outlined how a range of issues taken from the wider social context of oral health described in the previous chapter can impact upon dental work. It has been proposed that there should be a greater recognition of the contribution to achieving oral health made by informal health care workers. There are opportunities for greater cooperation between informal and formal health care workers, but the evidence would suggest that these opportunities are not being used to their best advantage. While everyone can be an informal health care worker, only some undergo the process of professional socialization required to become a formal health care worker. Formal oral health care work is stressful: a finding reciprocated by the large numbers of lay people who cite anxiety about treatment as a major barrier to accessing formal care.

Practice implications

- The realization that formal oral health care work is only one part of a much wider range of oral health activity can be challenging. Equally challenging for lay people is the contradictory situation they are placed in when entering a dental surgery, perhaps encountering a situation where they change from being an active person to a passive patient.
- If the lay person is to move from being passive to active in the dental surgery, there is a need for an increased professional investment in communication skills. The evidence at present is that there are deficiencies in communication with both adolescents and adults.
- There are several complementary aspects of access. Some of these aspects can be remedied within the organization of formal oral health care. There is evidence that there are substantial barriers to accessing this care which also have a negative impact upon the aim of achieving oral health.
- Poor communication with lay people is only one of several sources of stress that have the potential to generate a serious impact upon all members of the formal dental team.

References

Anderson, R. and Newman, J. (1973). Societal and individual determinants of medical care utilisation in the US. *Milbank Memorial Fund Quarterly*, **51**, 95–124.
Anderson, R. J. and Morgan, J. D. (1992). Marketing dentistry: a pilot study in Dudley. *Community Dent. Health*, **9**, supplement 1.
Arnbjerg, D., Soderfeldt, B., Palmqvist, S., et al. (1992). Factors determining satisfaction with dental care. *Community Dent. Health*, **9**, 295–300.
Ayer, W. A. and Corah, N. L. (1984). Behavioural factors influencing dental treatment. In *Social Sciences and Dentistry. A critical bibliography* (L. K. Cohen and P. S. Bryant, eds) pp. 267–322, London: Quintessence.
Baker, E., Israel, B. and Schurman, S. (1996). Role of control and support in occupational stress: an integrated model. *Soc. Sci. Med.*, **43**, 1145–1159.
Bauer, J. C. and Pierson, A. P. (1978). *Factors Which Affect the Utilisation of Dental*

Services. Maryland: US Department of Health Education and Welfare.

Banks, M., Beresford, S., Morell, D., Waller, J. and Watkins, C. (1975). Factors influencing demand for primary medical care among women aged 20–44 years. *Int. J. Epidemiol.*, **4**, 189–195.

Bosmajian, C. P. and Bosmajian, L. (1983). *Personalised Guide to Stress Evaluation*. London: Mosby.

Bradshaw, J. (1972). The concept of social need. *New Society*, **19**, 640–643.

Collett, H. (1969). Influence of dentist–patient relationships on attitudes and adjustments to dental treatment. *J. Am. Dent. Assoc.*, **79**: 879–884.

Cooper, C. L., Cooper, R. and Eaker, L. (1988). *Living With Stress*. London: Penguin.

Cooper, C. L., Watts, J. and Kelly, M. (1987). Job satisfaction, mental health and job stressors among general dental practitioners in the UK. *Br. Dent. J.*, **162**, 77–81.

Craven, R. C., Blinkhorn, A. and Roberts, C. (1995). A survey of job stress and job satisfaction among DSAs in the north-west of England. *Br. Dent. J.*, **178**, 101–104.

Croucher, R. (1989). *The Performance Gap. Patients' Views about Dental Care and the Prevention of Periodontal Disease*. Research Report 23. London: Health Education Authority.

Dean, G. (1969). The causes of death of South African doctors and dentists. *S. Afr. Med. J.*, **43**, 495–500.

DiMatteo, M. R., McBride, C. A., Shugars, D. A. and O'Neil, E. H. (1995). Public attitudes towards dentists: a U.S. household survey. *J. Am. Dent. Assoc.*, **126**, 1563–1570.

Eddie, S. (1984). Frequency of attendance in the general dental sevice in Scotland. *Br. Dent. J.*, **157**, 267–270.

Emling, R. C. (1980). Employee and patient management in times of stress. *Compen. Continu. Educ. Dent.*, **1**, 351–355.

Finch, H., Keegan, J., Ward, K., et al. (1988). *Barriers to the Receipt of Dental Care: A Qualitative Research Study*. London: Social and Community Planning Research.

Friedson, E. (1970). *Profession of Medicine*. New York: Dodd, Mead & Co.

Gerbert, B., Bleecker, T. and Saub, E. (1994). Dentists and the patients who love them: professional and patient views of dentistry. *Br. Dent. J.*, **177**, 287–291.

Gerhardt, U. (1989). *Ideas About Illness: An Intellectual and Political History of Medical Sociology*. Basingstoke: Macmillan.

Gerson, L. W. (1972). Expectations of 'sick role' exemptions for dental problems. *J. Can. Dent. Assoc.*, **38**, 370–372.

Godwin, W. C., Starks, D., Green, T. and Koran, A. (1981). Identification of sources of stress in practice by recent dental graduates. *J. Dent. Educ.*, **45**, 220–221.

Goedhart, H., Eijkman, M. A. J. and ter Horst, G. (1996). Quality of dental care: the view of regular attenders. *Community Dent. Oral Epidemiol.*, **24**, 28–31.

Goldstein, M. (1979). Sources of stress and interpersonal support among first year dental students. *J. Dent. Educ.*, **43**, 625–629.

Greenwood, M. (1993). Patients' views of oral day surgery. *Br. Dent. J.*, **175**, 130–132.

Health Education Authority (1996). *The Scientific Basis of Dental Health Education. A Policy Document*. London: Health Education Authority.

Hill, G. and Harvey, W. (1972). Mortality of dentists. *Br. Dent. J.*, **132**, 179–182.

Ireland, E. (1983). Dental practice burnout. *Compend. Continu. Educ. Dent.*, **4**, 367–369

Kasl, S. V. and Cobb, S. (1966). Health behaviour, illness behaviour and sick role behaviour. *Arch. Environ. Res.*, **12**, 246–247.

Kent, G. (1987). Stress amongst dentists. In *Stress in Health Professionals* (R. Payne and J. Firth-Cozens, eds.). Chichester: Wiley.

Kraemer, L. (1990). Impact of faculty and work role models on the professional socialization of dental hygienists. *J. Dent. Hygiene*, **64**, 278–285.

Lahti, S., Verkasalo, M., Hausen, H. and Tuutti, H. (1996). Ideal role behaviours as seen by dentists and patients themselves and by their role partners: do they differ? *Community Dent. Oral Epidemiol.*, **24**, 245–248.

Lim, C. S., Waite, I. M., Craft, M., Dickinson, J. and Croucher, R. (1984). An investigation into the response of subjects to a plaque control programme as influenced by friends and relatives. *J. Clin. Periodontol.*, **11**, 432–442.

Linn, E. L. (1971). Role behaviours in two dental clinics: a trial of Nadel's criteria. *Human Organisation*, **26**, 141–148.

Locker, D. (1989). *An Introduction to Behavioural Science and Dentistry*. London: Routledge.

Locker, D., Burman, D. and Otchere, D. (1989). Work-related stress and its predictors among Canadian dental assistants. *Community Dent. Oral Epidemiol.*, **17**, 263–266.

Locker, D. (1996). Work stress, job satisfaction and emotional well-being among Canadian dental assistants. *Community Dent. Oral Epidemiol.*, **24**, 133–137.

Maslach, C. (1982). *Burnout – the Cost of Caring*. New York: Prentice Hall.

Mellor, A. C. and Milgrom, P. (1995a). Prevalence of complaints by patients against general dental practitioners in Greater Manchester. *Br. Dent. J.*, **178**, 249–253.

Mellor, A. C. and Milgrom, P. (1995b). Dentists' attitudes towards frustrating patient visits: relationship to satisfaction and malpractice complaints. *Community Dent. Oral Epidemiol.*, **23**, 15–19.

Newton, J. T. and Gibbons, D. (1996) Stress in general practice: a qualitative comparison of dentists working within the NHS and those working within an independent capitation scheme. *Br. Dent. J.*, **180**, 329–334.

Osborne, D. and Croucher, R. (1994). Levels of burnout in general dental practitioners in the south-east of England. *Br. Dent. J.*, **177**, 372–377.

O'Mullane, D. and Robinson, M. (1984). The distribution of dentists and the uptake of dental treatment by schoolchildren in England. *Community Dent. Oral Epidemiol.*, **5**, 156–159.

O'Shea, R. M., Corah, N. and Ayer, W. (1984). Sources of dentists' stress. *J. Am. Dent. Assoc.* **109**, 48–51.

Parsons, T. (1951). *The Social System*. Glencoe: Free Press.

Penchansky, R. and Thomas, J. W. (1981). The concept of access. Definition and relationship to consumer satisfaction. *Med. Care*, **19**, 127–140.

Robinson, P., Zalrewska, J. M., Maini, M., et al. (1994). Dental visiting behaviour and experiences of men with HIV. *Br. Dent. J.*, **176**, 175–179.

Russek, H. (1962). Emotional stress and coronary heart disease in American physicians, dentists and lawyers. *Am. J. Med. Sci.*, **243**, 716–725.

Sachs, R., Zullo, T. and Close, J. (1981). Concerns of entering dental students. *J. Dent. Educ.*, **45**, 133–136.

Sheiham, A. and Croucher, R. (1994). Current perspectives on improving chairside dental health education for adults. *Int. Dent. J.*, **44**, 202–206.

Shuval, J. (1975). Socialization of health professionals in Israel: early sources of congruence and differentiation. *J. Med. Educ.*, **50**, 443–457.

Smith, T. Weinstein, P., Milgrem, P. and Getz, T. (1984). An evaluation of an institution-based dental fears clinic. *J. Dent. Res.*, **63**, 272–275.

Stacey, M. (1993). *The Sociology of Health and Healing*. London: Routledge.

Szasz, T. S. and Hollender, M. H. (1956). A contribution to the philosophy of medicine: the basic models of the doctor–patient relationship. *Arch. Intern. Med.*, **97**, 585–592.

Tisdelle, D. A., Hansen, D., St. Lawrence, J. and Brown, J. (1984). Stress management training for dental students. *J. Dent. Educ.*, **48**, 196–201.

Tuckett, D., Boulton, M., Olson, C., et al. (1985). *Meetings Between Experts*. London: Tavistock.
Todd, J. and Lader, D. (1991). *Adult Dental Health, 1988, UK*. London: HMSO.
Tudor–Hart, J. (1971). The Inverse Care Law. *Lancet*, i, 405–412.
Van Groenistijn, M. A. J., Maas-de Waal, C. J., Mileman, P. A. and Swallow, J. N. (1980). The ideal dentist. *Soc. Sci. Med.*, **14A**, 533–540.
Wadsworth, M. E. J., Butterfield, W. J. H. and Blaney, R. (1971). *Health and Sickness: The Choice of Treatment*. London: Tavistock.
Wanless, M. B. and Holloway, P. J. (1994). An analysis of audio-recordings of general dental practitioners' consultations with adolescent patients. *Br. Dent. J.*, **177**, 94–98.
Young, T. (1975). Questionnaire on the need for recusitation in the dental surgery. *Anaesthesia*, **30**, 391–401.
Zola, I. K. (1973). Pathways to the doctor: from person to patient. *Soc. Sci. Med.*, **7**, 677–689.

Chapter 4

Helping patients to achieve oral health

In the previous chapter we pointed out the distinction between illness behaviour and health behaviour. Illness behaviour refers to the steps that people take to treat disease, such as visiting a dentist to relieve a toothache. In this chapter, we turn to aspects of health behaviour, the actions that people take to maintain or improve health. Brushing, flossing and eating a low-sugar diet are attempts to achieve the positive definition of health suggested by the World Health Organization. Chairside dental health education (Sheiham and Croucher, 1994), which concerns the individual dentist, is crucial for meeting this aim.

Models of health behaviour

Psychologists and sociologists have developed several models or theories which can be used to explain why and when patients will put effort into achieving health. The Health Belief Model (HBM), developed by sociologists, holds that a person's views about his or her susceptibility to disease, the seriousness of the disease and the ability to avoid negative consequences are important. The Theory of Planned Behaviour, often used by psychologists, argues that attitudes are most important. The individual's and the community's attitudes to healthy behaviour combine with beliefs about ability to control health and illness to determine behaviour (McCaul et al., 1988; Tedesco et al., 1992; McGoldrick, 1997).

Although they have had some success, neither of these models has been particularly good at predicting how people will behave in the dental setting. Perhaps this is because different models are needed for different situations. For example, one model might be useful for understanding reactions to chronic illness, but another for acute disease. Another possibility is that most approaches have largely ignored the effects of social and situational factors. Someone might believe that a diet of sugar-free foods and regular flossing are important for oral health, but may not have the financial resources to purchase dental floss or relatively expensive sugar-free snacks.

The Stages of Change Model

One approach that has received increasing support over the past few years is the Stages of Change Model. It emphasizes two important aspects of behavioural change. One aspect is that change can be difficult. For example, stopping smoking or making large changes in diet can be hard to achieve, even for people who want to improve their health. Often, behaviour becomes habitual and a part of everyday routine, so that a significant change in lifestyle may be required. The second aspect emphasized by this model is that behavioural change is not a simple process. People rarely make a change before thinking about it first, perhaps preparing for the change, and then instituting it. In other words, a person may go through a number of stages before making and maintaining an alteration to his or her health behaviour.

Prochaska and DiClemente (1992) suggested that the process of change could be described in five stages as follows:

1. **The precontemplation stage.** Here, a person may be engaging in certain behaviour, such as eating many sugary snacks, and not considering changing this habit.
2. **The contemplation stage.** This is the stage when a person is thinking about a change, perhaps weighing up the pros and cons of eating a healthy diet.
3. **The preparation stage.** This occurs when a person has decided to make a change, and is preparing him- or herself for the new behaviour by making definite plans.
4. **The action stage.** After a person has prepared, the actual behaviour change is made.
5. **The maintenance stage.** Often it is important to work at maintaining a behavioural change. Many people who smoke find it relatively easy to quit for a few weeks or months, but many begin to smoke again, even after the body has overcome the physiological addiction.

Seeing behavioural change in this way makes it clear that the needs of different individuals will vary considerably. One person may need practical help in altering his lifestyle. He might have been thinking about how to make a change (i.e. is in the preparation stage) and requires practical assistance with how to achieve it. Perhaps he will ask for a demonstration on how to use dental floss. Another person might be in the maintenance stage. This individual might floss when she remembers, but may often forget. How could this person be helped to maintain her health behaviour? Yet a third person might be in the precontemplation stage, either not knowing about the importance of flossing or not believing in its importance.

It can be seen that these three people require different kinds of intervention. It is also possible to see that an intervention may serve to move a person from one stage to another. Although there may not be any obvious change in behaviour immediately, such a change is more likely in the long run if a dentist helps people to move through the stages.

Health promotion packages have generally focused on providing information to people. In the terms of the Stages of Change Model, the aim has been to move people from the precontemplation stage to the contemplation and preparation stages. The general aims of health promotion involve encouraging people to engage in health behaviour by (1) fostering awareness of its importance and (2) preparing the groundwork in the necessary ability and skills. Research on this educational aspect forms the basis of the next section of the chapter.

However, the Stages of Change Model suggests that educational material will not always result in behavioural change. Although education may be necessary, it may not always be sufficient. An individual may also need some motivation before engaging in the health behaviour. One basic difficulty with encouraging preventive care in any health area is that the consequences of unhealthy behaviour may not be experienced for many years. Often, a person is being asked to make an immediate sacrifice for health in the distant future. Children are most at risk because they are less likely than adults to be concerned with long-term objectives and less able to imagine the results of poor oral health habits. This chapter includes a section on how patients might be motivated to improve their oral hygiene behaviour.

The final section of the chapter provides an outline of a programme that brings together the educational and motivational approaches, both of which are necessary before behaviour is changed. The programme is one that individual dentists can use when attempting to improve the oral health of patients.

The educational approach

According to the Stages of Change Model, people will move out of the precontemplation stage only when they appreciate the importance of regular care and the meaning of symptoms. Several surveys have shown that there is a surprising lack of knowledge about hygiene practices in the general population. In one sample of dental patients, 63% reported that they had never heard of the word 'plaque', 29% could not remember having been instructed on how to brush their teeth, and none could remember having been told of the significance of the stickiness or frequency of eating sweets (Linn, 1974). In a study of mothers of preschool children, only 20% reported having received any advice on how to care for their children's teeth (Blinkhorn, 1978). Another survey of 16- to 20-year-olds indicated that 25% thought that it was 'natural' for their gums to bleed during brushing (Craft and Croucher, 1980). While it is important to realize that these results are based on respondents' memories (perhaps they had been told but had forgotten), these studies suggest that there is a significant lack of accurate information about dental care.

Experiments on educational programmes

There have been numerous attempts to improve knowledge and skills. The usual method has been to first select a sample of patients, randomly divide them into two groups, and then provide the education (perhaps through films or discussion) to one group but not to the other. The purpose of this random assignment is to ensure that any relevant variables, such as income level, social class or educational attainment, will be represented equally in the two groups.

Long-term effects of educational programmes

A good example of an experiment on dental education is given by Horowitz et al. (1976). One group of children was given 10 30-minute sessions on plaque removal, being taught in small groups by a dental hygienist. They were told about plaque, how to identify it with disclosing agents, and how to remove it. Each day for the next six months, plaque removal was practised under supervision. Disclosing agents were used regularly and the children were asked to rebrush and refloss any remaining plaque. All of this added up to a considerable amount of time, effort and education. The comparison group of children were not given any of this extra information or practice.

In this study, the investigators hoped that the educational intervention would improve the children's oral health. Three measures of oral hygiene were taken: a plaque score; a gingival inflammation (GI) score; and a caries score. These measures were taken before the programme began (called a baseline), again at the end of the treatment sessions (at eight months) and then again four months later.

At baseline, the two groups were similar on all measures, indicating that they were comparable to begin with. At the eight-month assessment there was a significant decline in GI scores in the education group compared with the control group. This was initially encouraging, but at 12 months there was again no difference. There was no long-term effect, and there were never any differences in caries levels or the amount of plaque in the two groups.

This is a typical result. The general finding of such studies has been short-term gain on plaque removal during the intervention but little improvement when further assessments are made several months later. It seems that people often revert to their previous behaviour when the intervention ceases. While educational programmes increase the amount of knowledge and skill that people possess, they have only a small effect on long-term behaviour (Kay and Locker, 1996).

Reasons for the failure of educational programmes to improve oral health
There are several possible reasons for the lack of long-term effects on health after educational interventions. One is that the programmes are usually work or school-centred: encouragement and practice may be given at school, but few attempts are made to integrate these into the home environment. This may be crucial. Perhaps, too, the people in such studies become dependent on the teaching staff to remind them to brush and floss. These programmes make little attempt to address the issue of maintenance: when the programme ends, so too do the constant reminders.

Another possibility is that while the educational approach provides part of the answer to changing behaviour, it is not in itself sufficient. Educational approaches might move some people up the series of stages, but not give them sufficient motivation or incentive to actually put their knowledge into action. Any discrepancy between what people know they should do and their actual behaviour may be due to motivational factors, especially the perceived consequences of their actions. This aspect of preventive care is discussed later in the chapter.

Education in practice
While educational programmes might not have a direct effect on oral health, they clearly improve knowledge and understanding. Misunderstandings are remarkably common between professionals and lay people, and often information is forgotten within minutes of the end of an interview. Because of this, there have been strong recommendations to provide patients with written information – something that they can take away to read over and remind themselves of the important points of a consultation. Many dentists display pamphlets in their waiting rooms, but there is a large body of

evidence that they are not understood by a substantial number of patients (Blinkhorn and Verity, 1979; Newton, 1995). Their usefulness also depends on whether they are noticed, read, believed and remembered (Ley, 1988).

Understanding text

Several factors need to be taken into account when designing educational material. Kanouse and Hayes-Roth (1980) list ways to increase the ease with which text can be understood. These include:

- Using active rather than passive verbs.
- Using concrete rather than abstract words.
- Stating ideas explicitly rather than implicitly.
- Using the same words consistently when referring to a disease or treatment.
- Using numbering when presenting facts.
- Putting old information at the beginning of a sentence, new information at the end.

The typeface is also important, as Poulton et al. (1970) point out. They provide several guidelines:

- Type size should be at least 10 point.
- Indenting the first line of a paragraph increases speed of reading.
- Printing in capital letters reduces speed of comprehension.
- Printing in italics reduces speed of reading.
- Headings will stand out better if they are in a typeface different from the text.
- Unjustified lines are easier to read.

Ease of reading

Another aspect of ease of comprehension is 'readability'. Text with a large proportion of polysyllabic words and long sentences is difficult to read. Short sentences are much easier. One way of calculating reading ease is to use the Flesch formula (Flesch, 1951):

$$\text{Reading ease} = 206.835 - 0.846 \; wl - 1.05 \; sl$$

where wl = number of syllables per 100 words (word length) and sl = number of words per sentence (sentence length).

A score below 60 is considered 'fairly difficult', below 50 'difficult'. For material designed for children, the score should be much higher, perhaps 90 plus.

As well as testing text for reading ease, it would also be important to select terms that could be understood by most readers. For example, the word 'plaque' is short but few people understand its meaning. If such terms are to be used, they need explanation.

Expertise
Not only must care be taken in deciding *what* is given to patients, but also in selecting *who* gives the information. Patients are more likely to accept and follow advice when it is given by someone whom they consider to be an expert, rather than by someone who is less qualified. This principle was tested by asking dentists, dental assistants and receptionists to give patients the same brief speech: 'There is a new dental care booklet I think you should read. It is free of charge if you just fill out this card with your name and address and drop it in a mail box'. Each card was covertly marked to indicate which of the three individuals gave the card to the patient. In one practice, 60% of the dentist's patients returned the card, 43% of the assistant's, and 23% of the receptionist's; in the other practice the rates were 47%, 27% and 13%, respectively (Levine et al., 1978). These results suggest that if a dental assistant or receptionist is to give advice, then the message may need to be reinforced in some way by the dentist.

The motivational approach

Many social scientists believe that educational approaches to preventive care must be complemented by increasing patients' motivation. In the terms of the Stages of Change Model, people will move from the contemplation and preparation stages to the action and maintenance stages only when they can see some kind of clear benefit for doing so. Furthermore, the benefit needs to be apparent in the short-term rather than some years in the future.

Behavioural analysis

The basic theory behind this approach is fairly straightforward. The likelihood that a person will behave in a certain way depends on the *consequences* of that behaviour. When someone performs an action and the consequences are rewarding, the person is likely to repeat that action again in the future. A dental student may study a subject either because it is intrinsically rewarding or because it is necessary to pass an examination in order to qualify, and qualification is rewarding. Conversely, the behaviour is less likely to be repeated if a person believes that the consequences of an action will be unfavourable. For example, a person may not begin to smoke cigarettes if he or she believes that it will have a negative effect on his or her health in the future. In both cases, the future consequences can be said to determine the present behaviour.

Reinforcement

Psychologists use the term 'reinforcement' to mean any consequence that increases the likelihood of behaviour. The reinforcement could be based on primary biological needs (e.g. food, water) or on things that are not intrinsically rewarding but have become so because of past experience (e.g. money), called secondary reinforcers. Another distinction is between positive and negative reinforcers. A positive reinforcer is a consequence that is pleasant and increases the likelihood of behaviour when it is offered. A dentist may work harder and see more patients if there is the promise of financial reward. An unpleasant event that can be avoided through some kind of action is called a negative reinforcer. The threat of failing an examination or being asked to leave a course of study are negative reinforcers. Faced with such consequences, a student may begin reading textbooks and studying in order to avoid them.

Punishment is quite a different concept. It is an unpleasant consequence which reduces the likelihood of behaviour being repeated. A parent who revokes a child's privileges for being naughty or a dentist who chastises a patient for eating too much sugar are both attempting, through punishment, to reduce the likelihood of these behaviours.

Applications of a behavioural analysis

These principles have been widely applied in psychology. As an example of how they might be used in practice, consider how a dentist might react to children in the surgery. A child who is well behaved and cooperative during treatment might be praised and given a small present such as a sticky badge. For this child, there is a positive consequence for attending and cooperating.

Preventive care

There are a large number of studies reporting the successful use of this principle of reinforcement in a wide variety of situations, including the encouragement of preventive care. Zifferblat (1975) argues that whether or not a patient follows advice is a function of the events that immediately precede and follow the prescribed behaviour. If a patient can feel or observe that 'this is the time to take

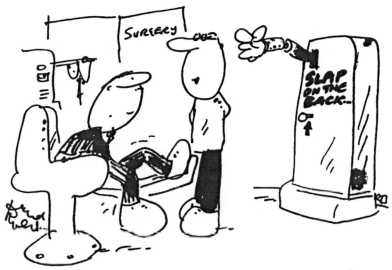

"You've been a splendid patient — stand by the machine and press the button..."
(Reproduced by permission of David Myers.)

my medication' or 'this is the time to brush and floss my teeth' easily
and unambiguously, compliance would tend to be high.

If, however, there is no obvious signal or negative consequences to
ignoring advice, compliance would be low. This could occur if a drug
or advice is given as a preventive measure: by the time the patient
realizes that the advice was important, it is already too late. A
problem that people have when on a diet is that the positive
consequences (weight loss) will be experienced sometime in the
future, while the negative consequences (hunger) are experienced in
the present.

There are similar difficulties for dental patients. While brushing
with a fluoride toothpaste, reducing sugar consumption and regular
flossing may reduce the likelihood of caries and periodontal disease in
the long run, noticeable symptoms may not appear for months or
years. The most important factor in caries development is diet,
particularly the amount and frequency of sugar consumption. Eating
sugar has positive short-term consequences while the negative
consequences are apparent only in the longer term.

From the behavioural analyst's point of view, prevention is
inherently problematic. Patients are being asked to act in order to
avoid disease, but this involves a sacrifice of an immediate reward for
dental health some time in the distant future.

Because brushing and dietary changes may not be inherently reinforcing, preventive care is unlikely if there is no external reason or motivation for compliance. There are two ways in which this difficulty might be overcome. One method is to provide positive reinforcements which are contingent on self-care: people are given rewards if they engage in health behaviour. This approach has formed the bulk of research in this area. The second method involves making the negative consequences of poor oral health care more salient. While this has always been one aim of educational programmes, there are additional strategies that can be used which are consistent with the motivational approach.

Providing positive reinforcements
This common-sense approach is used both by parents when praising their children for brushing and by dentists when congratulating their patients for looking after their teeth. However, a psychologist would require some experimental validation of this principle – some evidence that the procedure of providing external positive reinforcements for practising regular preventive measures is indeed useful. Does providing reinforcements improve preventive care?

Material incentives
In experiments with children and adults, rewards are often given in the form of material goods such as toys or money rather than verbal praise. For example, Reiss et al. (1976) attempted to encourage mothers to bring their children for a dental screening. These parents were from low-income families, so that cash seemed to be an appropriate incentive. One-third of the mothers received a note giving an explanation of the screening and a request to attend with their children. Another third received this note plus two personal calls, one on the telephone and one in person. The third group received the note plus a promise of $5.00 if they attended.

The results indicated that the cash incentive was the most effective of the three methods and was much more cost-effective than the two personal calls. In another study with children themselves, those who were given small rewards for having clean teeth improved their hygiene more over the course of the study than a control group of children who were not rewarded (Martens et al., 1973).

Although these and many other studies have indicated that this approach is effective, one concern about using material rewards is the possibility that once the incentives are withdrawn, the behaviour will return to previous levels or, worse, that it might cease altogether. Fortunately, there is evidence that this does not necessarily occur. In the case of the screening attendance study described above, more children in the reward group completed any necessary restorative work than in the other two groups, even though continued attendance was not rewarded financially. Similarly, in the study with children themselves, the difference between the control and incentive groups was maintained six months after the termination of the reward regime.

Providing material rewards can be rather expensive, so it would be useful to compare it with other methods for increasing motivation and preventive behaviour. Does reinforcement add to the effectiveness of education? This question was studied by dividing the patients of a dental practice into two groups (Iwata and Becksfort, 1981). One group was given an education programme about the detrimental effects of plaque, the importance of controlling it and the means of control. The patients' teeth were examined and cleaned, and disclosing tablets were issued so that the patients could monitor their plaque. On two later visits, further instruction and guided practice with brushing technique were given. A second group of patients was given this education programme plus an incentive: their treatment could cost up to 25% less if they were able to keep their plaque scores down.

At the end of the treatment programme, both groups of patients had lower plaque scores than at the beginning, indicating that both education alone and education plus incentive had an effect. However, the education plus incentive group showed a greater improvement: only one of 14 patients in the education-only group reduced their plaque by 10% or more while 15 of the 17 patients in the education plus incentive group did so. Furthermore, six months later the improvement for the incentive plus education group was maintained over the initial baseline level, but this was not the case for the education-alone group. Providing education plus an incentive was a more effective strategy than education alone.

Another study exploring the relative usefulness of various methods has been reported by Kegeles et al. (1978). Children were given a slide show about the aetiology of dental disease, health and cosmetic consequences of decay, and the effectiveness of fluoride as a preventive measure. They were then assigned to one of three groups. Those in one group were given no further attention, except that they were allowed to ask questions about the slide show. Those in the second group were given two discussion periods on the Health Belief Model, exploring ideas of seriousness, vulnerability and preventability. The children in the third group were offered some small cash incentives if they volunteered for and continued through the treatment programme.

Treatment was then offered to all three groups. It involved using a mouthrinse at home twice a day from a bottle which contained a 14-day supply. The bottles were designed so that the children could not simply dispose of the contents all at once: a stopper ensured that they would be ready for use only at six-hourly intervals. Every two weeks, the bottles were to be returned, and the next bottle picked up. This procedure continued for 20 weeks. The results indicated that the information plus incentive condition was again the most effective, as shown in Figure 4.1. For example, 49% of the children given an incentive picked up the last bottle, 31% of the information-only group and 18% of the discussion group children. That the discussion condition was the least effective is surprising, but a similar result was found in another study, in which the treatment involved topical fluoride applications (Lund et al., 1977).

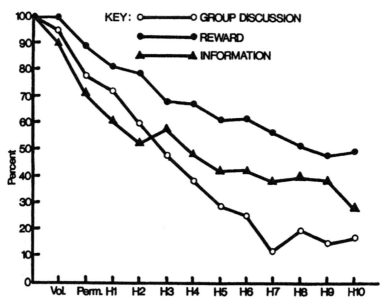

Figure 4.1. Percentages of children in each condition who complied with each stage of the mouthrinse programme. From Kegeles et al. (1978), with permission.

Problems with material reinforcements
These studies are unsatisfactory for a number of reasons. While they illustrate that positive reinforcement is effective, they also show that it does not work for everyone. Only half the children in the study by Kegeles et al. completed the whole programme. This may be because some of the children were in the precontemplation stage and the

rewards were not sufficient to change behaviour without understanding. The same reinforcement was offered to all children: perhaps
not everyone will be impressed by the same type of reward. Some
patients may prefer cash, but others may prefer toys or other age-
specific reinforcements. Another practical difficulty with these studies
is that the cost of the rewards could add up to a considerable sum if a
dentist were to offer them to all patients. There are several reports by
dentists who use 'star' systems. Patients are asked to keep a record
card, and every time a check-up is satisfactory, a star is added to it.
Bronze, silver or gold stars could be given, depending on the results.
Dentists have claimed that such inexpensive rewards are useful, but a
controlled study is required to evaluate the approach.

Another issue is that many of these studies portray patients as
passive recipients of reinforcements, seemingly being manipulated by
the psychologists or dentists. This portrayal may not correspond
particularly well to how we see ourselves or our relationships with
patients. Nor do these studies involve parents, who are important in
encouraging healthy dental habits in their children.

Involving parents in care
Every attempt should be made to encourage parental involvement
when attempting to change a child's health habits. It is equally
important that parents be helped to use positive reinforcement rather
than punishment, as illustrated by Claerhout and Lutzker (1981).
They identified four children (5–9 years of age) who presented
particular problems because of their lack of regular oral health care at
home. The children and the parents were invited to discuss the
problem and the parents expressed their willingness to become
involved. At first, the frequency of brushing was charted without
reinforcements being given. Each time the children brushed, a note
was made on a calendar. This provided some baseline data, indicating
to all concerned the exact nature of the problem. Snyder's test (which
measures the amount of lactobacilli in the mouth) and Greene's index
(for plaque) were also administered. Then, each time the children
brushed twice per day at home, they would be given a small
reinforcement by their parents.

The results of this intervention were excellent. It increased
brushing and had significant effects on lactobacilli and plaque scores.
Simply placing stars on a calendar was sufficient to increase brushing
from low baseline levels to almost 100% compliance for two children.
For the other two, small rewards were used: for example, once one
child had gained 20 stars for regular care, some pocket money was
given. The parents volunteered that they did not mind giving cash
reinforcements if this would help prevent serious future problems. An

interesting aspect of this programme was that the children were involved in choosing their own rewards: in one case the child chose her own supper menu one day a week. One year after the completion of the structured programme, the parents of these children were again contacted, and they reported that the oral hygiene practices continued to be satisfactory.

Thumb sucking

Thumb sucking can also be reduced by such methods. It often occurs at times of stress (Lauterbach, 1990) and can be seen as a way that children try to comfort themselves, so that sources of stress should be examined. De LaCruz and Geboy (1983) describe how they eliminated thumb sucking in an 8-year-old boy after various interventions had failed. The parents were asked to observe the child for an hour each day, charting the occasions when he was sucking his thumb. This indicated that he was thumb sucking about half the time. He was then told that if he could reduce his thumb sucking to about 25% of the time, he would be given a gold star for each day he accomplished this target. When he accumulated seven stars, he would be allowed to choose an inexpensive gift.

Within three weeks, thumb sucking was eliminated completely. After 27 days, the child suggested termination of the programme himself, because he no longer required it. Five months later, there was still no thumb sucking. A more thorough description of a similar procedure is given by Cripes et al. (1986).

Self-reinforcement

With adults, externally provided reinforcements may not be needed. They can be encouraged to reward themselves for performing health care tasks. They are capable of choosing their own reinforcements (e.g. a new pair of shoes or a favourite meal) and administering them correctly. One variant of this is called the Premack Principle. There are many actions in which people engage regularly: dressing in the morning, watering the house plants, watching television, and so on. These kinds of behaviour can act as reinforcers for other kinds of behaviour if they are sequenced correctly. For example, patients could be asked not to dress in the morning until they have brushed their teeth, or not to watch television before flossing.

Modelling

People's behaviour depends not only on the consequences of their own actions but also on observing the consequences of *others'* behaviour. A dental student, for example, will learn much by watching how a qualified dentist talks with patients or goes about a restoration. If the restoration goes well, the student is likely to repeat the dentist's actions when practising him- or herself. Similarly, if a student observes a dentist talking to a patient in a way that results in open and successful communication, he or she might later repeat such behaviour. On the other hand, if the patient becomes upset, the student may decide to treat patients differently. In other words, the teaching staff provide a model for the student, indicating which behaviour could be expected to have positive or negative consequences.

Modelling can have deleterious effects. One of the problems that medical educators have in changing smoking habits, for example, is that many smokers can cite examples of friends or relatives who smoked all their lives with few ill-effects. Similarly, many people can cite examples of others who rarely visit the dentist yet seem to have healthy teeth and gums.

Modelling can also be used to change behaviour in more positive directions, and it can be used in everyday dental practice. For example, when one child has a check-up which is satisfactory or better than the previous one, this could be rewarded in the presence of siblings. By seeing a brother or sister rewarded for good or improving hygiene, other members of a family may also be encouraged to take better care of their teeth and gums.

Highlighting negative consequences

Another possible method of increasing the likelihood of preventive care would be to provide negative reinforcements: those which increase the likelihood of behaviour when they are removed. In order for decay or extractions to be negatively reinforcing in themselves, it would be necessary for people to consider these possibilities as consequences to be avoided. However, this does not seem to be the case for many people. In one survey, only 10% of those interviewed thought that dental problems would have a significant effect on their job, appearance or social life.

Walsh et al. (1985) used gingival bleeding as a negative reinforcer. Patients were taught that bleeding was a sign of disease and that it could be avoided by increased self-care. Patients who were given this information showed a significant improvement in gingival health; a result which was not found for a control group of patients.

Disclosing agents
These agents are often used as one part of a preventive programme, and for this reason it is difficult to disentangle their effects from other aspects of the educational and motivational packages. For example, in

an experiment by Clark et al. (1973), children were presented with a traditional education programme on the problems that could be expected to result from poor dental hygiene. Information about the ways in which these problems could be overcome was given in two different ways. For half of the children, instruction on flossing and brushing and the use of disclosing tablets was given in a lecture. Afterwards, they were given kits that included a supply of disclosing tablets and two toothbrushes. For the other half, the instruction was given personally. These children's teeth were stained and then examined for plaque by a dental hygienist and by other members of the group. Those showing plaque were given assistance in brushing and flossing. Furthermore, over the next eight months, once a week, a dental assistant supervised the staining, flossing and brushing of teeth. Six months after the completion of the supervision, all the children's teeth were again stained and measures taken. For the children in the group given the education programme alone, there was no change in the amount of debris on the teeth, but for those given specific and continuing instruction, a highly significant reduction in plaque was found.

Some conclusions may be drawn from this study. Since both groups of children were given disclosing agents, they alone could not have been responsible for the difference. Further, since there was no improvement for the first group, it seems unlikely that simply issuing disclosing tablets to patients will improve hygiene (although they may halt further deterioration — it was not possible to tell here without another control group). Other conclusions are more difficult to draw. Indeed, it is difficult to specify just what was responsible for the difference in plaque scores, because there were several differences in procedure between the two groups. The students in the supervised group were instructed to examine each other's teeth, so that the disclosing agent made plaque visible not only for the individual concerned but also for others: the condition of one's teeth became public knowledge. Perhaps it was this public disclosure that was important. It also seems probable that the dental hygienist was rewarding, through praise, those children whose plaque scores were improving. It may not have been the disclosing agent *per se* that was important, but rather the assistant's positive reactions to the state of the children's teeth.

Disclosing agents do seem to be effective in informing patients about the state of their oral hygiene, particularly if photographs are used (Albino et al., 1977), but they may be useful in changing behaviour only if the plaque that they show is considered to have some negative connotation. Simply issuing them to patients and hoping for the best is unlikely to be effective.

Punishment

Punishment is an unpleasant consequence which reduces the likelihood of behaviour being repeated. While punishment is effective in the short run, it seems to have few long-term effects: once the threat is no longer present, the behaviour often returns. There are also several problems with using punishment in a professional capacity. Not the least of these is ethical: does the dentist have the right to judge patients and their behaviour? The use of punishment has several connotations for patients, implying as it does that the dentist is in a position of power and authority over them. There may also be some doubt as to which behaviour will be reduced. For example, a patient may have a highly cariogenic diet because he sucks sugary mints throughout the day. Reprimanding the patient may curtail the consumption of mints, but conversely, the patient may decide to change his dentist to one who offers practical advice on non-cariogenic substitutes.

For these reasons, psychologists tend not to use punishment. Rather, they would look for instances of desirable behaviour and positively reinforce these. This was the method used with the young boy who was sucking his thumb, discussed earlier. Instead of reprimanding him when he was thumb sucking, his parents provided positive reinforcement when he was not engaging in this behaviour. Similarly, if the aims were to change dietary habits, the procedure would be to praise the consumption of non-sugary foods rather than to punish the eating of sweets. It is most likely that there will be some aspects of a patient's behaviour that are consistent with good oral health, and these should be positively reinforced.

Designing a preventive programme

It must be said at the outset that a dentist who hopes to make large and clinically significant changes in most patients' behaviour is likely to be disappointed. It is very difficult to accomplish this in the few minutes a year that is available for most patients. This is partly because for most patients, oral health will not have the same priority as it will for a dentist, and partly because it is difficult to change habitual patterns of behaviour. Results from one survey showed that over 40% of adults admitted they had not changed their hygiene habits after being given instructions by their dentists, but on the other hand, 50% of the sample claimed that they did make some changes, even if they were minimal. Some changed to a particular design of toothbrush, for example. The challenge of preventive dentistry is to increase the likelihood of change and to ensure that it is maintained in the future.

In order to be effective, several ground rules must be followed when applying the principle of reinforcement explained in this chapter. Most of the six steps outlined below have been discussed previously, but this section provides a working summary that could be useful for practising dentists.

1. A clear and precise definition of the problem

Many people are unaware of the basic facts and do not have the required skills needed for adequate prevention. As discussed earlier, it is important that verbal advice is supplemented by written material whenever possible. It is equally important that patients are able to understand and remember this information. A detailed assessment may be needed so that gaps in knowledge and skills may be identified and filled.

In order to change behaviour, it is important to specify exactly what requires alteration. To say that a patient has 'poor dental health' is not adequate, since this is too global and vague a definition and could be due to many different factors. More specific behavioural definitions are needed, since patients must know which of their health care patterns need to be changed. A thorough inspection will highlight the major health problem. For example, if a patient has severe gingivitis, this suggests that brushing and flossing must be improved. The presence of new carious lesions indicates the consumption of many cariogenic snacks and drinks, so diet needs attention.

2. Monitoring the frequency of the problem behaviour

Once the broad nature of the specific difficulty is identified, it is important to gain some information about current behaviour. Making a record of current behaviour serves three purposes. First, a chart provides both the patient and the dentist with information about the scope of the problem. This helps to define it. Second, it serves as a baseline, so a patient is able to see that he or she is making progress in future attempts to change. This can have beneficial effects in itself. Third, charting provides the dentist with a way of monitoring the effectiveness of the preventive programme. Although it is unlikely that the chart will be completely accurate, if a baseline is gathered before an intervention begins, progress can be checked.

To give a practical example, a patient visits the dentist with many cavities which will require several appointments to restore. The problem seems to be that the patient consumes cariogenic foods at frequent intervals throughout the day. In order to gauge the exact frequency of this behaviour, the patient could be asked to place a tick on a prepared sheet each time sugar is eaten. The range of foods that contain sugar would need to be explained. The patient might also be asked to indicate the circumstances in which this occurs – the antecedents. Over a period of one or two weeks before the next appointment, the patient will be able to see – and perhaps be surprised at – the amount and timing of sugar consumption. It may be more effective if the dentist provides a chart rather than leaving it to the patient. An example is shown in Table 4.1.

Table 4.1. An example of a chart that could be used to monitor the frequency and circumstances of eating sugary foods. The patient indicates whenever a sugary food is eaten. In order to find out what triggers this behaviour, the circumstances (e.g. during morning coffee) are also noted

Date _____

Time	Circumstances
08:00–09:00	
09:00–10:00	
10:00–11:00	
11:00–12:00	
.	
.	
.	

3. Specifying the aims of the intervention

Just as it is important to specify the nature of the problem, so too is it important to consider what the dentist and patient aim to achieve. This is called the *target* behaviour. For a patient who eats five sugary snacks a day, the aim might be to reduce this to one per day. For someone who never flosses, the aim might be to floss thoroughly twice a week at specific times.

4. Changing the behaviour

However, these overall targets may not be achieved easily. Research has shown that it is very difficult to make major changes to patients' habits. Requesting someone to make an abrupt and extensive change in diet, for example, is unlikely to have any effect, but it is possible to change small aspects of behaviour one at a time, so that over a long period considerable improvements can be made. By taking realistically small steps, which the patient can reasonably be expected to achieve, the ultimate goal can be reached.

Shaping

The procedure that is used to accomplish this is called *shaping*. Horner and Keilitz (1975) describe how they used shaping in order to teach patients with severe learning difficulties to brush their teeth. While brushing is relatively easy for most people, it involves a complex series of behaviours which can be a formidable task for people with learning disabilities. In shaping, the steps needed in order to attain a final goal are noted. Then each of these steps is reinforced in turn until the whole series is learned.

In order to ascertain exactly what behaviours are involved in tooth brushing, Horner and Keilitz first videotaped a competent person brushing his teeth. From this tape, they identified several small steps:

1. Pick up and hold the toothbrush.
2. Wet the toothbrush.
3. Remove cap of toothpaste.
4. Apply toothpaste to brush.
5. Replace cap on the toothpaste.
Steps 6–11 involved brushing various parts of the mouth.
12. Rinse the toothbrush.
13. Rinse the sink.
14. Put equipment away.
15. Discard any paper cups or tissue used.

The teaching of each of these steps was accomplished by giving rewards. When a patient picked up and held the toothbrush, for example, he was praised or given tokens that could be exchanged for sugarless gum. When this learning was accomplished, the next step was taught: rewards were given only when the toothbrush was wetted. These two pieces of behaviour were then *chained* together so that a reward was given only when the patient both picked up the toothbrush and wetted it. Then the next step was taught. This procedure was followed until the whole series of actions could be accomplished. Brushing one's teeth might form only a small part of an overall programme of self-care which might also include such skills as dressing, eating with utensils, and so on.

Brushing

A similar procedure of rewarding small pieces of behaviour, one at a time, can be used for teaching children to brush their teeth. Accepted wisdom has it that children do not have the necessary motor skills to brush their teeth adequately until they are 7 or 8 years of age, but Poche et al. (1982) showed that children aged between three and four years can learn to brush competently. In their study, tooth brushing was broken down into 16 steps, representing the cleaning of different parts of the mouth. At each step, the children were required to hold the brush at a 45° angle and to use a soft scrubbing motion. Before training, the children were able to perform only about 9% of the necessary actions, but afterwards they were able to accomplish 96% of the necessary actions. At an eight-week follow-up, 87% of the steps were performed. This increased ability also resulted in a decrease in plaque levels. Thus, this study suggests that young children do have the necessary motor skills but that they may require more detailed training than older children.

Dietary changes

Similarly, diet can be altered. The aim would be to reduce sugar intake slowly. If, at baseline, a patient was having five cariogenic snacks per day, the first step might be to cut this down to four. When this has been accomplished, some reinforcement would be given and the next step would be to reduce this to three, and so on. During this time, the patient would continue to chart eating habits and bring the charts to each dental appointment. At the same time, an alternative behaviour could be encouraged: instead of eating sugary foods, sugarless gum could be substituted. The frequency of this behaviour would also be monitored and reinforced.

5. Reinforcement

The consequences of any change in behaviour should always be made clear. There is the praise and encouragement of the dentist but, as mentioned earlier in the chapter, most people are quite capable of reinforcing themselves. Once a certain level of sugar intake has been achieved, patients could reinforce themselves with a new coat or a day trip somewhere — whatever they find rewarding. Over the next few weeks, a lower sugar intake would be required before the reinforcement was given, and so on.

Reinforcements should be provided as soon as possible after the desired behaviour. In part, simply marking a chart or calendar serves this purpose since the patient can see some positive consequence of the behaviour. This feedback can itself be useful encouragement. Immediate reinforcement is particularly important for children, who will be less likely than adults to appreciate a link between brushing on Monday and a trip to see a film on Saturday. Here, the involvement of parents is crucial since only they are in a position to dispense a reinforcement immediately after brushing. The frequency with which reinforcements are given should decrease as time goes on, particularly after the target behaviour is reached. The ultimate aim is to integrate oral health habits into a patient's everyday activities so that they become habitual.

6. Failures in preventive programmes

It would be misleading to suggest that the educational and motivational approaches advocated in this chapter would be helpful to all patients, and for this reason it is important for dentists to monitor patients' progress. There are several reasons why such a programme could fail. Perhaps a patient is not yet in the action stage, the chosen reinforcement is not appropriate or sufficiently enticing, or the patient is not comfortable with rewarding him- or herself: further encouragement may be required. Another possibility concerns lack of support from parent or spouse. Programmes where other members of the family are involved typically have much higher success rates than those which concentrate solely on the patient.

Motivation
Motivation might be a problem. Weinstein et al. (1983) argue that 'When the patient does not desire to change, or does not perceive that a problem worth acting on exists, there is little a practitioner can do' (p. 68). Syrjala et al. (1994) have developed a questionnaire that measures the extent to which a patient is intrinsically or extrinsically motivated. People who are extrinsically motivated and who agree with such statements as 'I don't think dental diseases are very important' or 'My teeth decay in spite of brushing' may require a different approach from those who are intrinsically motivated. Similarly, Nuttall (1996) has developed a scale to measure dental indifference, or the extent to which people are reluctant to implement preventive dental intervention. Motivation can be increased by asking the patient to make a list of the reasons why the behaviour should change. Stressing the importance of physical appearance might be very useful in this respect.

A related problem is that of commitment. Although a patient may indicate that he or she intends to follow a programme, these good intentions may not be translated into behaviour. One method for increasing commitment is termed 'contracting'. Although it may seem rather artificial, it has proved to be an effective approach. The patient is asked to sign a form, such as that shown in Table 4.2, which is a 'public' commitment to the programme. In some studies, patients have been asked to deposit a sum of money, which would be returned only if they complete the programme: an especially successful method.

Table 4.2. A possible contract for monitoring sugar consumption

Before my appointment on _____

I agree to:
1. Carry the chart with me whenever I am likely to eat a snack
2. Tick the chart each time I eat a snack containing sugar
3. Consider what it could be doing to my teeth
4. Bring the chart to my next appointment

Signed _____ Date_____

The staff's role
Other reasons why a preventive programme might not succeed concerns the views of staff. There are two possibilities here. One is that the dentist or other staff might have reservations about implementing the programme consistently and enthusiastically. It may seem that patients are being manipulated in some way. This is not the aim. Rather, it is to maximize the probability that patients will engage in dental health behaviours and find the consequences of this behaviour rewarding. The staff's role is to instigate and support the programme, but the final responsibility for its effectiveness is the patient's. Since staff are unlikely to be able to discuss dental problems with a patient for more than a few minutes per year, it is important that the maximum benefit be gained from these interviews.

The other possibility is that the programme is instituted mechanically, without due concern for the interpersonal aspects of the situation. The way that staff relate to patients is often more important than what they advise. While information is, of course, necessary, it may well be less critical than patients' feelings that they are being cared for and understood.

The social context
Another possible reason why a preventive programme may fail is the

patient's social context. There may be a lack of support from a spouse or parent. Although every patient's social context needs to be taken into account, perhaps the most problematic is the child's social world. Cariogenic foods are very important for children, not simply because they are inherently pleasant to eat, but also because they form part of the social system of exchange. The sharing of sugary foods provides an important means of reaffirming friendships and gaining status. From a child's point of view, the everyday contingencies of the playground may be much more compelling than those of the occasional visit to the dentist. The replacement of cariogenic with non-cariogenic foods may be possible, but the social cost to the child must be considered.

Summary

Several models have been developed to explain why some people are more likely to engage in health behaviour than others. The Stages of Change Model postulates that people move through a series of stages, from not being aware that there is a difficulty that could be addressed through to taking definite actions and maintaining these actions. One reason why many people neglect their oral health may be a lack of knowledge and skills. Educational programmes have had little direct effect on oral health, but they do increase knowledge. Several methods can be used to improve home care. One possibility is providing positive reinforcement, either directly through inexpensive rewards or indirectly through modelling. Other members of the family can be involved in such programmes and patients can be shown how to monitor and reinforce their own behaviour. The aim is to integrate new patterns of dental care within the habitual routines of everyday life. People can also be helped to appreciate and avoid the negative consequences of neglect. Whatever the method used, it is important that the required changes are specified very clearly and precisely and that these changes are made slowly in small and realistic steps.

Practice implications

- Different patients are likely to be at different stages in the process of changing behaviour.
- Dental practitioners are in a good position to remedy any lack of knowledge but it is important to make individual assessments and tailor information according to a patient's ability to

understand.
- Written information is a useful memory aid.
- When attempting to change behaviour, use positive reinforcements rather than reprimands.
- Changing habits is difficult and time-consuming. Don't try to do too much at once and accept that, despite your best efforts, it will not be possible to change the behaviour of all patients.

Suggested reading

For a more thorough discussion of psychological principles applied to transmitting information, see Ley, P. (1988). *Communicating with Patients*. London: Croom Helm. For preventive dental care, see Weinstein, P., Getz, T. and Milgrom, P. (1991). *Oral Self-care: Strategies for Preventive Dentistry*. Seattle: University of Washington.

References

Albino, J., Julian, D. and Slakter, M. (1977). Effects of an instructional programme on plaque and gingivitis in adolescents. *J. Public Health Dent.*, **37**, 281–289.

Blinkhorn, A. (1978). Influence of social norms on toothbrushing behaviour of pre-school children. *Community Dent. Oral Epidemiol.*, **6**, 222–226.

Blinkhorn, A. and Verity, J. (1979). Assessment of the readability of dental health education literature. *Community Dent. Oral Epidemiol.*, **7**, 195–198.

Cripes, M., Miraglia, M. and Gaulin-Kremer, E. (1986). Monitoring and reinforcement to eliminate thumbsucking. *J. Dent. Child.*, **53**, 48–52.

Claerhout, S. and Lutzker, J. (1981). Increasing children's self-initiated compliance to dental regimes. *Behav. Ther.*, **12**, 165–176.

Clark, C., Fintz, J. and Elwell, K. (1973). Eliminating dental plaque in the sixth grade. *J. Public Health Dent.*, **33**, 70–74.

Craft, M. and Croucher, R. (1980). *The 16 to 20 Study*. London: Health Education Council.

De LaCruz, M. and Geboy, M. (1983). Elimination of thumbsucking through contingency management. *J. Dent. Child.*, **50**, 39–41.

Flesch, R. P. (1951). *How to Test Readability*. New York: Harper & Row.

Horner, R. and Keilitz, I. (1975). Training mentally retarded adolescents to brush their teeth. *J. Appl. Behav. Anal.*, **8**, 301–309.

Horowitz, A., Suomi, J., Peterson, J., et al. (1976). Effects of supervised daily dental plaque removal by children. *J. Public Health Dent.*, **36**, 193–200.

Iwata, B. and Becksfort, C. (1981). Behavioural research in preventive dentistry. *J. Appl. Behav. Anal.*, **14**, 111–120.

Kanouse, D. and Hayes-Roth, B. (1980). Cognitive considerations in the design of product warnings. In *Banbury Report 6: Product labelling and health risks*. (L. A. Morris, M. Mazzio and I. Barofsky, eds) New York: Cold Spring Harbor Laboratories.

Kay, E. and Locker, D. (1996). Is health education effective? A systematic review of current evidence. *Community Dent. Oral Epidemiol.*, **24**, 231–235.

Kegeles, S., Lund, A. and Weisenberg, M. (1978). Acceptance by children of a daily home mouthrinse programme. *Soc. Sci. Med.*, **12**, 199–210.

Lauterbach, W. (1990). Stimulus-response (S-R) questions for identifying the function of problem behaviour: the example of thumb sucking. *Br. J. Clin. Psychol.*, **29**, 51–57.

Levine, B., Moss, K., Ramsey, P., et al. (1978). Patient compliance with advice as a function of communicator expertise. *J. Soc. Psychol.*, **104**, 309–310.

Ley, P. (1988). *Communicating with Patients*. London: Croom Helm.

Linn, E. (1974). What dental patients don't know about dental care. *J. Public Health Dent.*, **34**, 39–41.

Lund, A., Kegeles, S. and Weisenberg, M. (1977). Motivational techniques for increasing acceptance of preventive health measures. *Med. Care*, **15**, 678–692.

McCaul, K., O'Neill, H. and Glasgow, R. (1988). Predicting the performance of dental hygiene behaviours: an examination of the Fishbein and Ajzen Model and self-efficacy expectations. *J Appl. Soc. Psychol.*, **18**, 114–128.

McGoldrick, P. (1997). Principles of health behaviour and health education. In *Community Oral Health* (C. Pine, ed.) London: Butterworth.

Martens, L., Frazier, P., Kirt, K., et al. (1973). Developing brushing performance in second graders through behaviour modification. *Health Serv. Rep.*, **88**, 818–823.

Newton, J. (1995). The readability and utility of general dental practice patient information leaflets: an evaluation. *Br. Dent. J.*, **178**, 329–332.

Nuttall, N. (1996). Initial development of a scale to measure dental indifference. *Community Dent. Oral Epidemiol.*, **24**, 112–116.

Poche, C., McCubbrey, H. and Munn, T. (1982). The development of correct toothbrushing technique. *J. Appl. Behav. Anal.*, **15**, 315–320.

Poulton, E., Warren, T. and Bond, J. (1970). Ergonomics in journal design. *Applied Ergonomics*, **13**, 207–209.

Prochaska, J. and DiClemete, C. (1992). Stages of change in the modification of problem behaviours. In *Progress in Behaviour Modification* (M. Hersen, R. Eiser and P. Miller, eds) Newbury Park: Sage.

Reiss, M., Piotrowski, W. and Bailey, J. (1976). Behavioural community psychology: encouraging low income parents to seek dental care for their children. *J. Appl. Behav. Anal.*, **9**, 387–397.

Sheiham, A. and Croucher, R. (1994). Current perspectives on improving chairside dental health education for adults. *Int. Dent. J.*, **44**, 202–206.

Syrjala, A., Knuuttila, M. and Syrjala, L. (1994). Obstacles to regular dental care related to extrinsic and intrinsic motivation. *Community Dent. Oral Epidemiol.*, **22**, 269–272.

Tedesco, L., Keffer, M., Davis, E. and Christersson, L. (1992). Effect of a social cognitive intervention on oral health status, behavior reports and cognitions. *J. Periodontol.*, **63**, 567–575.

Walsh, M., Heckman, B. and Moreau-Diettinger, R. (1985). Use of gingival bleeding for reinforcement of oral home care behaviour. *Community Dent. Oral Epidemiol.*, **13**, 133–135.

Weinstein P., Getz, T. and Milgrom, R. (1983). Oral self-care: a promising alternative behavior model. *J. Am. Dent. Assoc.*, **107**, 67–70.

Ziflerblat, S. M. (1975). Increasing patient compliance through the applied analysis of behaviour. *Prev. Med.*, **4**, 173–182.

Chapter 5

The nature and causes of anxiety

Anxiety experienced by dental patients is of concern, partly because of its effects on patients and partly because of its effects on dentists themselves. Depending on how it is measured, 3–5% of the general population can be said to have a debilitatingly high level of fear of dentistry (Hakeberg et al., 1992; Moore et al., 1993). There seems little doubt that patients' anxiety can interfere with dental care. Surveys typically show that a sizeable proportion of the general population avoid making regular visits to the dentist because they are 'too frightened' to do so. In a survey of 6000 people, 43% reported that they avoided going to the dentist unless they were experiencing trouble with their teeth (Todd and Walker, 1980). Of these, 58% said that part of the reason was that they were 'scared of the dentist' (Todd et al., 1982). Further evidence that anxiety contributes to delay in visiting the dentist is provided by Curson and Coplans (1970). When they interviewed 100 patients in an emergency clinic, 38% said that they did not make regular visits because they were too afraid of the experience. Of these, only 12% made and kept further appointments for a course of treatment at the clinic: a result similar to the findings of other studies (Stewart et al., 1994).

Such results have several implications for dental practitioners. On the one hand, they mean that dentists will encounter some patients who require extensive restorative work, yet will not agree to have it done. On the other hand, anxious patients can present personal and interpersonal problems. For dentists who consider themselves as professionals who wish to help patients and improve their quality of life, it can be disturbing to be seen as someone who inflicts distress. The first section of this chapter provides an outline of the nature of anxiety. This is useful in understanding its aetiology, a topic discussed in the second half of the chapter. Methods of alleviating anxiety are discussed in Chapter 6.

The nature of anxiety

The term 'anxiety' has been used in several ways by psychologists. For some, anxiety is a 'vague, unpleasant feeling accompanied by a premonition that something undesirable is about to happen' (Kagan and Havemann, 1976). This is primarily a subjective definition, relying on how people feel. Sometimes a distinction is made between anxiety and fear: anxiety is said to be a general feeling of discomfort, while fear is considered to be a reaction to a specific event or object. For example, a person might be anxious about a visit to the dentist and specifically fearful about an extraction. Often the words anxiety and fear are used interchangeably, however, and no distinction will be made here.

Many psychologists use a three-component model to understand anxiety. In the studies discussed in this chapter, subjective, behavioural and physiological measures have been used. A behavioural measure often includes avoidance of the dentist; physiological measures include heart rate and sweating, while self-report measures include verbal or written expressions of distress. However, these three types of measures may not correspond to each other. On a behavioural measure of avoidance, for example, a patient who attends a dentist regularly might not be considered anxious, yet he or she might express worry or concern. Conversely, someone may refuse to see a dentist yet deny any suggestion of anxiety. Rather than debate which kind of measure is the most valid, in recent years psychologists have tended to consider all three as components of anxiety, reflecting different aspects of the problem. Some researchers have examined how different situations evoke anxiety, others have concentrated on subjective reports, while yet others have explored physiological and behavioural components.

The situation

Intuitively, some situations are more anxiety-provoking than others. It would be useful to specify which dental procedures are associated with the most anxiety. Wardle (1982a) asked patients attending a dental hospital to rate how anxious they would feel if they had to undergo each of a list of procedures. The patients were asked to indicate if they would be 'not anxious', 'slightly anxious', 'fairly anxious', 'very anxious' or 'extremely anxious' for each procedure. Extraction led the list, followed by injection and drilling. Polishing was the least feared. Similar results have been found with other groups, as shown in Table 5.1 (Gale, 1972). Here, a longer list of procedures was given but the general order is similar to Wardle's results.

Table 5.1 makes an important point. The amount of fear that a person experiences cannot be specified from knowledge of the situation alone. The patients were divided into high- and low-fear groups according to their overall feelings about visiting the dentist. The rankings of the procedures for the two groups were virtually identical (a correlation of 0.98 where a perfect correlation would equal 1.0). Although there was much agreement about the relative stressfulness of the various procedures, there were also important individual differences in the amount of anxiety that each one provoked.

Table 5.1. Ranking of dental situations from the most feared to the least feared for high-fear and low-fear groups

Situation	Low-fear group	High-fear group
Dentist is pulling your tooth	1	2
Dentist is drilling your tooth	2	1
Dentist tells you that you have bad teeth	3	3
Dentist holds the syringe and needle in front of you	4	6
Dentist is giving you a shot	5	4
Having a probe placed in a cavity	6	5
.		
.		
.		
.		
Thinking about going to the dentist	15	12
Dentist cleans your teeth with steel probe	14	16
Getting in your car to go to the dentist	16	15
Dentist looks at your chart	17	17
.		
.		
.		
.		
Dentist asks you to rinse your mouth	24	24
Dentist tells you he is through	25	25

After Gale (1972), with permission.

All of the people involved in these studies were dental patients. Do other people see the problems in the same way? Jackson (1978) gave a longer list of 60 items to several different groups – dentists, hygienists, dental students, dental patients and dental phobics – and asked them to rank the items for their 'stressfulness'. Some items were ranked higher than others for all groups: 'Dentist is giving you a shot' and 'Having a root canal done' are two examples of high-stress items. However, there were some important differences in how the various groups ranked the items overall. Patients said that 'Dentist squirts water into your mouth' and 'Dentist prepares a shot of novocaine' were more stressful than did the dentists and hygienists. A particularly interesting finding concerned the rankings of the dental phobics: they found anticipating the dental visit (e.g. 'Getting into your car to go to the dentist' and 'Sitting in the dentist's waiting room') more stressful than did most of the other groups.

Other indications that it is not necessarily the drilling and filling that patients find frightening comes from studies of patients who are scheduled to see dental hygienists (de Jongh and Stouthard, 1993) or who are edentulous (Stouthard and Hoogstraten, 1990). Their levels of anxiety can also be high.

These findings indicate that the amount of fear a person experiences cannot be specified from knowledge of the type of treatment alone. Although there is much agreement between patients about the relative stressfulness of various procedures, there are also important individual differences in the amount of fear each one provokes. Thus it is important and useful to have standard ways of measuring how anxious each individual feels.

Self-reports of anxiety

Questionnaires can be used to measure the amount of anxiety a person experiences. Some of these questionnaires can be used in a variety of situations: the same one could be used whether the person is about to see a dentist, take a university examination or make a parachute jump. Other questionnaires are specific to certain settings in that they ask people how they feel about particular experiences, such as surgery or dentistry.

A general measure of anxiety

One popular method of measuring anxiety which can be used in many settings is the State–Trait Anxiety Inventory (STAI) developed by Speilberger et al. (1983). Speilberger makes a distinction between anxiety as a general personality trait and anxiety as a response to a particular situation. The former is known as *trait* anxiety. People with high trait anxiety are those whose feelings of personal adequacy and worth are threatened by a wide variety of circumstances, particularly where some kind of failure is a possibility. *State* anxiety, in contrast, is more transient, depending not so much on stable personality characteristics as on the specific situation. This type of anxiety varies as a function of the stresses that impinge on a person at a particular time. High state anxiety is evoked when an individual perceives a situation as threatening to physical or emotional well-being.

The STAI consists of 40 statements: 20 are designed to measure trait anxiety, while the other 20 measure state anxiety. An example of a trait item is 'I lack self-confidence', and an individual chooses one of four alternatives (almost never, sometimes, often or almost always) which best describes his or her feelings. In measuring state anxiety, the individual is asked to respond according to how he or she feels at the moment. For example, the item 'I feel calm' could be given one of the following four responses: not at all, somewhat, moderately so or very much so.

The STAI has been used extensively in dental research. Measures of state anxiety are particularly informative. Scores on these items of the STAI typically rise before a visit and then fall sharply afterwards. As discussed in the next chapter, state anxiety can be reduced considerably with short-term minimal interventions. The measurement of trait anxiety can also be informative. Wardle (1982a) gave her patients the trait anxiety items from the STAI while they were waiting for treatment at a dental hospital. She also took a number of physiological measures, finding a significant relationship between trait anxiety and the number of signs of physiological arousal that the patients were experiencing, such as sweatiness of the hands and dryness of the mouth.

Measuring dental anxiety

Besides questionnaires such as the STAI, which can be used in many situations, there are several questionnaires that have been designed specifically to measure anxiety in the dental setting. In order to arrive at the rankings shown in Table 5.1, patients were asked to indicate on a seven-point scale between 'no fear' and 'terror' their degree of fear about each of the procedures mentioned.

Another questionnaire is the Dental Anxiety Scale (DAS) developed by Corah (1969), shown in Table 5.2. Patients are asked to circle the alternative that best represents how they feel. Each alternative is given a simple numerical value from 1 to 5, so that a total score could range from 4 to 20. A score of 13–14 should alert the dentist, and patients with a score of 15 or more are almost always highly anxious (Corah et al., 1978). Although the DAS has been widely used, Humphris et al. (1995) have argued that one important weakness of the scale is that it does not include an item about fear of injections, and they have modified the DAS to include this.

Kleinknecht et al. (1973) have developed another approach, asking patients about their anxieties to a total of 27 specific items, such as making an appointment, seeing the needle and hearing the drill. Patients are asked to rate their fearfulness on a 1–5 scale, from 'none' to 'great' for each situation. This method provides a more precise view of a patient's fears than does Corah's DAS: detailed information which might be useful when attempting to alleviate the problem. These researchers have, however, found that responses to one question ('Generally, how fearful are you of dentistry?') correlate 0.89 with responses to all the other items (Kleinknecht and Bernstein, 1978), suggesting that this might be a useful question for preliminary screening of patients.

Table 5.2. The Dental Anxiety Scale

---

1. If you had to go to the dentist tomorrow, how would you feel about it?
   (a) I would look forward to it as a reasonably enjoyable experience
   (b) I wouldn't care one way or the other
   (c) I would be a little uneasy about it
   (d) I would be afraid that it would be unpleasant and painful
   (e) I would be very frightened of what the dentist might do

2. When you are waiting in the dentist's office for your turn in the chair, how do you feel?
   (a) Relaxed
   (b) A little uneasy
   (c) Tense
   (d) Anxious
   (e) So anxious that I sometimes break out in a sweat or almost feel physically sick

3. When you are in the dentist's chair while he gets his drill ready to begin working on your teeth, how do you feel? (Same alternatives as number 2)

4. You are in the dentist's chair to have your teeth cleaned. While you are waiting and the dentist is getting out the instruments which he will use to scrape your teeth around the gums, how do you feel? (Same alternatives as number 2)

From Corah (1969), with permission.

A method for assessing anxiety in children is shown in Figure 5.1. Venham (1979) asked the children in his study to choose which of the two alternatives on each of the eight cards best represented how they felt. A measure of anxiety was provided by totalling the number of times a child picked the cartoon depicting distress of some kind.

Validity of questionnaires
Instruments that aim to measure anxiety (or indeed any psychological factor) must fulfil certain conditions. An important requirement is that they can be shown to be valid, i.e. they must measure what they purport to measure. This can be shown in several ways. For example, scores on the state anxiety items of the STAI would be expected to

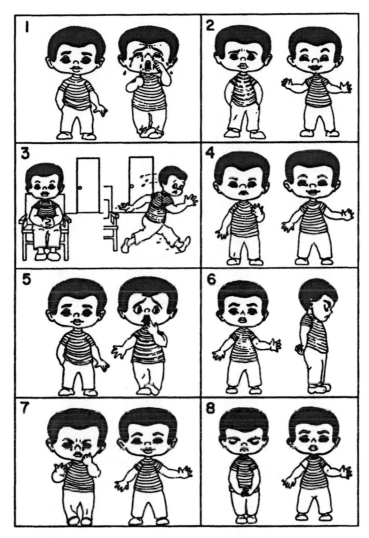

Figure 5.1. A method for assessing anxiety in children. Children are asked to indicate which drawing from each pair illustrates how they feel. From Venham (1979), with permission.

be different before and after a person undergoes a stressful experience. Also, we would expect higher levels of anxiety before an invasive procedure, such as a restoration, than before a check-up. This has been demonstrated in a study on dental patients (Tullman et al., 1979). All were attending the dentist on a regular basis, but the patients in one group were due to have only check-ups while the patients in the other group were scheduled for treatment, such as restoration. While they were waiting to see the dentist, all patients were given the state anxiety questionnaire to complete. As expected, the patients waiting for restorations reported higher anxiety than those waiting for check-ups. When given the questionnaire at the completion of the appointment, the treatment patients showed a significant decrease. At this point, the anxiety reported by the two groups was similar. These results show that the STAI state anxiety scale is sensitive to differences in the situation.

Another method of validating self-report questionnaires is to take physiological and behavioural measures and relate these to subjective feelings. People who have a high pulse rate at the dental surgery or who avoid attending whenever possible should score higher on self-report measures than those whose pulse rate is slower or who make regular visits. Corah used dentists' ratings of patient anxiety to validate his DAS. He first asked patients to fill out the questionnaire and then asked dentists to rate the patients' anxiety without knowing their responses on the scale. He found a significant relationship between these scores, indicating some validity.

Reliability of questionnaires

It is also important to investigate the reliability of these questionnaires. Test–retest reliability is tested by asking the same group of people to fill out the questionnaire on two occasions, some months apart. If very different answers are given at these two times, it means that the questionnaire is measuring a transient feeling rather than longer term anxiety. When Corah (1969) did this with the DAS at a three-month interval, he found a good correlation between the two scores ($r = 0.82$), indicating that the reliability of this questionnaire is high.

The questionnaires mentioned here have been shown to have adequate validity and reliability (Schuurs and Hoogstraten, 1993). Even though the different questionnaires may have given slightly different results (Locker et al., 1996), they can be used with some confidence by a researcher or a dentist who wishes to measure subjective anxiety. It also means that the effectiveness of methods that aim to alleviate anxiety can be tested by giving such questionnaires before and after an intervention. An investigator can then judge whether the intervention has made a difference to patients' subjective feelings.

The cognitive side of anxiety

These questionnaires can provide a useful measure of a patient's level of anxiety. However, another important way of gauging fear is to ask patients what they think about while in the chair or in the waiting room. Highly anxious patients often dwell upon the worst possible outcomes they can imagine, thinking, for example, that the appointment is likely to result in intense pain, or that the dentist will discover that there is a vast amount of work needed (de Jongh et al., 1994). This kind of 'catastrophic' thinking can be connected to a hypersensitivity to danger signs in the environment. An anxious patient may be very vigilant to any indication of threat such as the sight or sound of the drill, the wearing of a mask, or comments passed between members of the dental team. de Jongh et al. (1995) have developed the Dental Cognitions Questionnaire, which contains such items as 'The needle will break off', 'They will find something terribly wrong with me' and 'They might drill too deep'. Patients are asked to indicate both the frequency and the believability of the statements. A simple question, such as 'What do you think about when you are sitting in the dental chair?' could be a very useful question to gauge a patient's cognitions.

Physiological arousal

Another component of anxiety involves such autonomic signs as a higher pulse rate, dryness of the mouth and the release of stress hormones. Simpson et al. (1974) provide an illustration of how physiological variables are related to dental stress. Electrodes were placed on the forearms of children when they arrived for their first dental visit. After taking baseline measures before each child saw the dentist, they monitored changes in heart rate and galvanic skin responses to various procedures. The results for the children's heart rates are shown in Table 5.3. When the dentist changed into his white coat, for instance, the children's average heart rate increased by 10 beats per minute over baseline and it was 12 beats per minute higher when the dental chair was raised. When the examination was finished, their hearts were beating an average of 3 beats per minute below baseline.

The direction of the relationship between physiological arousal and subjective feelings of anxiety is far from clear. There is disagreement among psychologists as to whether arousal is a cause of feelings of anxiety or a response to them. Some psychologists argue that people first find that their hearts are racing and that they are perspiring, and then interpret these symptoms as signs of anxiety. Other psychologists contend that it is the other way around: that physiological arousal is a consequence of cognitions. A person may interpret a situation as being threatening and this then results in physiological arousal, perhaps through adrenaline and catecholamine release. Another problem is that few physiological signs are specific to particular emotions, in that the same signs might be shown for anger or exertion as for anxiety. In the dental chair, physiological arousal could be interpreted as anxiety, while on the sports field, it would be seen as a sign of exertion.

Table 5.3. Average changes in heart rate from baseline in the dental setting in children visiting for the first time

Activity	Changes in heart rate (beats/minute)
Dentist changes into a white coat	+10
Statement: 'I am a dentist'	+15
Elevation of dental chair	+12
Adjustment of lamp	+10
Intra-oral examination	−1
End of examination	−3

From Simpson et al. (1974), with permission.

Behaviour

A final component of anxiety is motor behaviour, which can take several forms. Behaviour problems shown by children (e.g. pushing the instruments away, refusing to open the mouth) are sometimes considered to be manifestations of anxiety. One method for assessing the amount of disruptive behaviour in children is a four-point scale developed by Frankl et al. (1962). A child is placed in one of four categories according to the following criteria:

1. **Definitely negative:** refusal of treatment, over-resistance and hostility, extreme fear, forceful crying, and massive withdrawal or isolation or both.
2. **Slightly negative:** minor negativism or resistance and minimal to moderate reserved fear, nervousness or crying.
3. **Slightly positive:** cautious acceptance of treatment, but with some reluctance, questions or delaying tactics; moderate willingness to comply with dentist.
4. **Definitely positive:** good rapport and appropriate verbal contact with operator, no sign of fear, interested in procedures.

It is preferable to be more precise than this. Melamed et al. (1975) listed a large number of behaviours which were considered to be fear-induced reactions to the dental surgery, as shown in Table 5.4. Instead of categorizing children on the basis of an overall impression, as Frankl did, Melamed et al. clearly specified which reactions they would include and time-sampled their occurrence. Every three minutes, the researcher indicated whether each of these had occurred. A child who was crying at any point during every three-minute interval would be given a higher score than someone who cried only once or twice. Each reaction was also weighted (as shown by the numbers in parentheses on the far left of Table 5.4), such that kicking the legs was scored as indicating twice as much anxiety as closing the eyes. In these ways, a more precise description of the children's behaviour was gained.

Table 5.4. Some of the items used for indicating the occurrence of fear-induced behaviour

Situation	Successive three-minute observation periods									
	1	2	3	4	5	6	7	8	9	10
Separation from mother										
(3) Cries										
(4) Clings to mother										
(4) Refuses to leave mother										
(5) Bodily carried in										
Office behaviour										
(1) Choking										
(2) Won't sit back										
(2) Attempts to dislodge instruments										
(2) Verbal complaints										
(2) Over-reaction to pain										
(2) White knuckles										
(2) Eyes closed										
(3) Cries at injection										
(3) Refuses to open mouth										
(3) Rigid posture										
(3) Crying										
(3) Dentist uses loud voice										
(4) Restraints used										
(4) Kicks										
(5) Dislodges instruments										
(5) Refuses to sit in chair										
(5) Leaves chair										

From Melamed et al. (1975), with permission.

Inter-observer agreement

Whenever such behavioural rating scales are used, it is important that there be a high level of agreement between observers. Such agreement is certainly not to be taken for granted, since different people will use different criteria and place different weightings on these. This problem is common whenever people's judgements are made. For example, Ludwick et al. (1964) were interested in comparing the quality of restorations undertaken by dentists and operating ancillaries in the US Navy. In order to do this, they asked experienced dentists to examine 152 restorations from the two groups, classifying them as excellent, good, fair or unsatisfactory. However, there was much disagreement between the seven dentists: in only 4% of the cases was there unanimous agreement, while in 9% the judgements ranged from excellent to poor. Incidentally, the same might be said about assessments of dental students' work. In one study (Naitkin and Guild, 1967), there was much inconsistency between assessors when assigning grades. Sometimes the same grade was assigned for very different reasons.

Similar problems apply when rating levels of anxiety. One observer might use very different criteria for what constitutes 'rigid posture' or 'dentist uses a loud voice' from another observer. In order to reduce this problem, at least two observers should be used in psychological studies. Before the study begins, they would make some observations and then compare notes. Through discussion, they can specify where they disagree and ensure that they would use the same criteria.

Avoidance of the dentist

There is evidence that fear of dentistry affects appointment-keeping and attendance on a regular basis (Stewart et al., 1994). Wardle (1982a) found a higher anxiety level in the patients who had not been to the dentist within the previous two years than those who attended within this time. It is possible to see how this could build up in a circular fashion: the longer a person delays visiting a dentist, the more likely it becomes that restorative work will be needed, thus raising the anxiety level of that person (Moore et al., 1991).

A good way to assess the impact of anxiety on attendance would be to give a questionnaire to patients before they were due to attend and then see if they turn up. When Kleinknecht and Bernstein (1978) used this method, they found support for the notion that anxiety affects attendance. Of those patients who had previously reported low fear, only 8% either cancelled or failed to show, while 24% of the high-fear patients missed their scheduled appointments.

Phobias

Some people have inordinately intense fears of particular situations, so much so that they will avoid contact at almost any cost. Such intense fears, called phobias, seem to be out of all proportion to the actual threat and do not respond to reason. The potential effects of such fears has been illustrated by Lautch (1971), who found that phobic patients suffered pain for an average of 17.3 days before consulting a dentist, compared with only 3.0 days for a matched sample of non-phobics. Such suffering is not uncommon: Segal (1986) reported that 15% of the patients attending an emergency clinic had been in pain for one month or more.

According to the American Psychiatric Association (1995) the following five criteria need to be met for this diagnosis:

A. Marked and persistent fear that is excessive or unreasonable, cued by the presence or anticipation of a specific object or situation.
B. Exposure to the phobic stimulus almost invariably provokes an immediate anxiety response.
C. The person recognizes that the fear is excessive or unreasonable.
D. The phobic situation(s) is (are) avoided or else endured with intense anxiety.
E. The avoidance, anxious anticipation or distress in the feared situation interfere significantly with the person's normal routine, occupational functioning or social activities or relationships, or there is marked distress about having the phobia.

The extent to which high levels of anxiety can affect the quality of patients' lives (criterion E) has been shown by Berggren (1993), who questioned patients who had been referred to a dental anxiety clinic. Over half indicated that their dental fear caused problems with social activities (eating out, meeting friends), 46% with going on vacation and 41% family relationships. Kent et al. (1996) designed a scale to measure the social and psychological effects of phobias. Phobic patients were likely to endorse items that indicated social and cognitive consequences (e.g. 'I feel that people will laugh at me if I tell them about my fears about dentistry' and 'The need to see a dentist is constantly on my mind'), avoidance (e.g. 'When walking or driving somewhere I take a route in order to avoid passing by a dentist's office' and 'I become upset when I see adverts on TV about tooth decay and tooth loss') and social inhibitions (e.g. 'I stop myself from smiling or I cover my mouth when I laugh' and 'I am reluctant to meet new people because of the state of my teeth').

Implications

These various components of anxiety are interdependent, but it is important to reiterate that there is no one-to-one relationship between them. One person who feels extremely anxious about dentistry may nevertheless attend regularly and be cooperative, while another person could be very disruptive. An illustration of this independence has been provided by a study in which heart rate recordings of children were taken while they were seated in the dental chair. Many of the children clenched their fists or forearms during examination, but for them there was no corresponding increase in heart rate. For more than one-third of the children, heart rate actually decreased during such behavioural displays of anxiety (Rosenberg and Katcher, 1976).

That these components of anxiety do not always correlate has several implications. One of these is theoretical, in that it is important, in studying anxiety, to take several measures sampling these different components. A practical implication for dental practitioners is that they may find it difficult to judge patients' feelings from their behaviour. It may be remembered that when validating his DAS, Corah correlated patients' responses on the DAS with dentists' judgements of their anxiety. Although the correlations were statistically significant, indicating some validity, they were fairly low, about 0.42. This means that the dentists' judgements and the patients' self-reports were often dissimilar.

A second implication concerns the decision about how to help. Two patients may report that they feel anxious, but for one, the main problem may seem to be behavioural (e.g. non-attendance), while for the other it may be physiological (e.g. a racing heart). Perhaps the former patient would benefit from a different intervention from the latter, as discussed in the next chapter.

The causes of anxiety

One of the more obvious answers to the question of why people are anxious about dental treatment is that they anticipate some suffering. Wardle (1982a) asked her patients about the amount of pain they anticipated from several dental procedures (e.g. extraction, drilling, polishing). She also asked them about the amount of anxiety they felt about these procedures and then correlated the two scores together:

most of the correlations were high (ranging from 0.65 to 0.85). Seventy-six per cent of the patients reporting high anxiety said that fear of pain was all or part of the reason for their fear. These and other results suggest that a central reason for dental anxiety is anticipated pain.

However, this does not provide a full understanding of dental anxiety. First, it does not explain why many people who expect to experience pain do not report anxiety. In Wardle's study, 70% of the fearful patients expected their treatment to be painful, but so too did 46% of the fearless patients. Furthermore, this explanation assumes that anxiety is a result of pain, either expected or experienced, such that pain leads to anxiety. Another possible explanation of this relationship is that anxiety leads to pain. Or perhaps the relationship is circular, so that anxiety leads to pain leads to anxiety, and so on.

There are some studies that support the possibility that heightened anxiety can affect pain tolerance and pain threshold. Kleinknecht and Bernstein (1978) posted anxiety questionnaires to patients before they arrived at the surgery. After the appointments, they asked the patients to indicate how much pain they had experienced during their treatment. When the high- and low-fear groups were compared, the high-fear patients reported more pain than the low-fear patients. This was not due to the types of treatment procedures the groups underwent, since these were similar. In some instances, at least, pain can be seen as a result or a symptom of anxiety rather than its cause.

In this section of the chapter, four main lines of research on the causes of anxiety are considered: 'preparedness'; uncertainty; negative experiences; and biological differences.

Preparedness

A first approach to the aetiology of anxiety involves the possibility that people are innately predisposed to become anxious about certain types of situations. Epidemiological studies of the sources of anxiety indicate that people are much more likely to develop anxieties and phobias about approaching spiders, cats and dogs than approaching many other situations. Many people are also frightened of being in an enclosed space. Although these animals and situations do not pose a realistic threat to well-being, many people find them difficult to tolerate. By contrast, phobias about some objectively dangerous situations are rare. For example, few people are phobic about travelling at high speeds on the roads, which poses a realistic threat.

One way of making sense of these findings is to suggest that people are innately 'prepared' to be fearful about and avoid objects which, in our evolutionary past, did pose a threat. Perhaps small animals carried a threat of disease, and enclosed spaces may have been associated with being trapped. Evolution could have favoured 'anxious genes' because anxiety may have raised the chances of survival. Since we are not prepared in the same way to be anxious about travelling at 70 m.p.h., such a phobia is rare (de Silva, 1988).

It is possible to see a link with dentistry. Lying on one's back with an adult placing sharp instruments in the mouth should in some sense be frightening. In particular, anxiety might be heightened if the adult is a stranger (patients often find the prospect of joining a new practice distressing because they are concerned that the dentist will have a 'rough manner'), or if the patient is a child (where there is a large disparity of strength). This idea goes some way towards explaining the widespread occurrence of dental anxiety.

Uncertainty

Anxiety is sometimes characterized as 'fear of the unknown' and there are indications from laboratory experiments in psychology that uncertainty, itself, is anxiety-provoking. Epstein and Roupenian (1970) persuaded people to volunteer for an experiment which involved undergoing a series of unpleasant electric shocks. Some were told that the probability of receiving a shock on any one trial was 1 in 20, while others were told that the chances were 19 in 20. On the basis of common sense, one would expect that the second group would be more anxious than the first, since their probability of receiving a nasty shock was much higher. In fact, the opposite occurred: on measures of skin conductance and heart rate, the 1 in 20 group showed higher anxiety than the 19 in 20 group. It seemed that those in the high-probability group resigned themselves to the pain, while those in the low-probability group could neither resign themselves nor dismiss the thought that the shock would occur.

That this kind of process might be operating in anxious dental patients was suggested by Wardle (1982b), who reported that many of the patients who she interviewed expected some kind of pain to occur. If they did not feel any discomfort on one visit, they would leave with the feeling that they had somehow got away with it. 'Any time now, he will get the nerve, and then it will really hurt' was a common thought reported by these patients when they underwent treatment. The probability of pain might be low, but it could happen at any time and therefore could not be dismissed. It is the *perceived* risk of pain, not necessarily the actual experience, that is important here. Although non-anxious patients typically make accurate predictions of the amount of pain they are likely to experience during invasive procedures, anxious patients usually overestimate the likelihood of discomfort (Arntz et al., 1990).

Previous learning

A third approach to the aetiology of dental anxiety involves learning processes. The contention here is that anxious patients have had some kind of previous experience which has led them to expect that dental care involves pain. The typical procedure used to study this possibility has involved first dividing patients into high- and low-anxiety groups. This may be done by questionnaire, by interviewing people about their feelings, or by direct observation of behaviour. The next step is to attempt to find differences in the experiences of these two groups of patients. Shaw (1975), for example, selected 100 anxious and 100 non-anxious children on the basis of their dentists' judgements of anxiety. On questioning the mothers of these children, she found that the anxious children were more likely to have had an extraction on their first visit to the dentist, many of them finding the experience traumatic. Similarly, Lautch (1971) interviewed phobic and non-phobic patients about their previous experiences. In his sample of 34 phobics, all reported at least one previous traumatic experience with a dentist, while only 10 of the 34 non-phobics could remember such an incident. Of the phobic patients who had returned to the dentist at least once after the experience (30 patients), all reported further traumas but only one of the non-phobics did so.

Classical conditioning

One way in which dental anxiety could be learned is through a process termed 'classical conditioning'. The early development of classical conditioning theory was due to Pavlov, a Russian physiologist working at the beginning of the twentieth century. In his original studies, he was interested in the digestive system, using dogs as his subjects. While giving food to his animals he noticed that after several feedings they would begin salivating *before* they tasted the food. Sometimes their digestive systems would begin to work at the sight of the handler who fed them. The animals had learned, on the basis of past experience, that there was an association between the sight of the food and actually tasting it.

Pavlov began experimenting with this phenomenon, presenting lights or tones to the animals whenever they were fed. After several pairings of food and light, for example, the dogs would begin salivating in response to the light alone, in the absence of food. The light could then be paired with a tone and then this, too, would elicit salivation. He hypothesized that there could be many such associations between biologically significant events (e.g. food, water) and neutral stimuli in the environment, and that this could account for much of human learning.

While psychologists today would consider this an oversimplification and would place more emphasis on other kinds of learning, there are several indications that classical conditioning is important in the learning of fears and anxiety. That it can be used to explain some fears has been demonstrated by Watson and Raynor (1920). In a much-quoted experiment, they showed a young child, named Albert, a white rat. At first, Albert seemed very interested in the rat and wanted to play with it. Then, Watson and Raynor paired a loud aversive noise (a hammer striking a steel bar) with each presentation of the rat, so that every time Albert saw or touched it he would also hear the unpleasant noise. After only six pairings, Albert began to be distressed at the sight of the rat in the absence of the noise. The notion that dental anxiety is the result of a classically conditioned association between pain and dental care has been supported many times (ter Horst and de Wit, 1993; Milgrom et al., 1995).

At first sight, these studies suggest that previous direct experience is an important cause of anxiety, but caution is required before making this conclusion. An important difficulty in most studies on the aetiology of anxiety is that investigators rely on the respondents' *memories* for information. Perhaps people who are anxious are more likely to recall negative experiences. Another possibility is that people are more likely to *interpret* an experience as negative if they are already anxious.

A further difficulty with this explanation is that in other studies of intensely fearful patients, not all patients have been able to remember traumatic incidents, suggesting that other kinds of experience are important for some people. Indeed, in the Shaw study, many of the children who were anxious about extractions and restorations had no history of a traumatic event. Furthermore, some children who have never been to the dentist are anxious on their first visit.

Generalization
It may be that fears about dentistry sometimes develop as a result of experiences in other settings. A patient might have been fearful when visiting a doctor (someone else who gives injections and who wears a white coat), and this fear could generalize to the dental setting. There was some supporting evidence for this kind of learning in Shaw's (1975) sample of dentally anxious children. In another report involving these same children (Semet, 1974), significantly more of the anxious children had a history of hospital admissions and negative attitudes towards the care they were given in hospital. It seemed as though their experiences with medical care *generalized* to dentistry.

Gale and Ayre (1969) illustrate how fears can generalize in odd and surprising ways. They describe one patient who was very frightened of the dental chair and who later became frightened of the chairs in hairdressers. In the case of Albert and the white rat, his distress generalized to other white furry objects, such as a white rabbit, cotton wool and a fur coat.

Anxiety and attendance patterns
In fact, there is no simple or clear relationship between previous experiences and anxiety. Brown et al. (1986) found that a DMFT (decayed/missing/filled teeth) index was negatively related to self-reports of anxiety: children with the greatest experience with invasive procedures had the lowest levels of anxiety. A similar pattern was found by Murray et al. (1989), who performed a particularly interesting longitudinal study. They analysed the dental records for children over a three-year period and found that frequency of attendance was an important factor. Children who attended irregularly and who received some invasive procedure during that time showed an increase in anxiety, while the anxiety levels for those who attended regularly and had such a procedure did not change. But children who did not receive any invasive treatment, whether or not they attended regularly, were the most anxious overall. The suggestion from both these and other studies (Davey, 1989) is that receiving invasive treatment in the context of regular attendance can act prophylactically. Clearly, more longitudinal studies are needed (Neverlien, 1994).

The family's anxiety
For some people, the learning involved in dental anxiety may have been more indirect, depending on the experiences of other people. Shoben and Borland (1954) and Fogione and Clarke (1974) were able to uncover a pattern of family experiences not limited to anxious patients themselves. In a fearful group of patients, there was a more unfavourable attitude towards dentistry among the patients' relatives and more reports of traumas experienced by these relatives. This result was replicated by Shaw, who also found that mothers of anxious children were themselves more anxious and were more likely to comment on previous distressing experiences. It may be that the anxious patients' relatives served as models, displaying to them the kinds of consequence they could expect from a visit to the dentist.

Evidence for the importance of this factor comes from a number of studies (Johnson and Baldwin, 1968; Klingberg et al., 1993; Corkey and Freeman, 1994). Johnson and Baldwin first gave the mothers of their young patients an anxiety scale to complete. They then made observations of the children while they were in the dental chair, rating their behaviour as being generally positive or negative. The results are shown in Table 5.5. Those mothers whose anxiety was high were more likely to have children who reacted negatively. Most of the children in the study were visiting the dentist for the first time, so their behaviour could not have been due to direct experience.

Table 5.5. The number of children showing positive or negative behaviour in the dentist's chair as related to their mothers' anxiety scores

Mothers' anxiety score	Children's behaviour rating	
	Positive	Negative
High	4	25
Low	25	6

From Johnson and Baldwin (1968), with permission.

A subsequent study (Koenigsberg and Johnson, 1972) showed that the relationship between mothers' anxiety and children's behaviour held for the first visit (which was for examination) but not for subsequent ones (for restorations). It seemed that actual experience became more significant for the children rather quickly. While some studies have replicated the relationship between mothers' anxiety and children's behaviour, there are also some failures to replicate (Bailey et al., 1973; Klorman et al., 1979), indicating that this particular association can be weak.

The dentist's role

Bernstein et al. (1979) examined the role of previous experience in a slightly different way. They first divided university students into high- and low-fear groups on the basis of their answers to a dental anxiety questionnaire. The students were then asked to write an essay describing their visits to the dentist as children. These essays were to include 'the features and events associated with those visits which determine present attitudes'. Forty-two per cent of the high-fear group mentioned pain during early appointments as a factor in their present reactions to dentistry, compared with 17.4% of the low-fear students. While these proportions discriminated between the groups to some extent, there was still the 58% of high-fear students who did not cite pain as a factor, and a sizeable minority of low-fear students who did experience pain.

This overlap could be clarified by considering another variable: the personality of the dentist. Half of the high-fear group mentioned negative behaviour on the part of the dentist as a factor in their feelings about dentistry, most of these students not citing pain as a reason at all. The dentists were considered 'impersonal', 'uncaring', 'disinterested' or 'cold'. It was about equally likely that an uncaring dentist was seen by the students as the reason for their feelings as was experience of pain. Furthermore, of the low-fear group who had experienced pain as children, many found the dentist 'careful', 'patient' and 'friendly'. The effects of the pain seemed to have been mitigated by a caring and concerned dentist. This study suggests that the dentist had an independent effect on the students' feelings (i.e. cold or disinterested behaviour was enough to make some students feel negatively about dentistry) and an interactive effect (i.e. caring and warmth could obviate the long-term effects of early painful experiences).

Thus, previous learning can take many forms. Experiences with pain may be important in developing anxiety about visits to the dentist, but the relationship between past experience and current anxiety is very complex. Fear can also generalize from one setting to others that appear similar in some way, so that a traumatic experience in a medical setting may generalize to dentistry. Other factors, such as attendance pattern and encounters with dentists who were seen as uncaring and unfriendly, can modify the meaning of a painful visit. In many cases, the learning may have occurred more indirectly. A patient's friends and relatives provide models, giving expectations about how much discomfort a person might feel at the dentist's surgery.

Biological differences

Another approach to the aetiology of anxiety involves the possibility that some people are more predisposed to become anxious or to learn anxiety responses than others because of innate biological variations. Biological differences could affect dental anxiety in the case of those people who have a lower pain threshold or lower pain tolerance than others. This could result in a greater likelihood of pain having been experienced in the past and thus higher anxiety about experiencing it in the future. Another possibility relates to the classical conditioning approach. Pavlov's work was based on a biological viewpoint, stressing the importance of physiological responses to environmental stimuli. Since arousal is an important component of anxiety, it may be that individual differences in anxiety are due to differences in 'arousability'.

Neuroticism

Research on the relationship between physiological activity and personality characteristics has been conducted by Hans Eysenck. One of the characteristics he uses in describing people is called Neuroticism, a term which has come to have many unfortunate connotations. People who answer in the affirmative to such questions as 'Are you moody?' and 'Do you often feel fed up?' would score high on the Neuroticism scale of the Eysenck Personality Questionnaire (EPQ). Eysenck argues that personality is firmly based on innate, genetically determined mechanisms. People who score high on the Neuroticism scale are said to have autonomic systems which, once aroused, persist in a high state of arousal for long periods. This could result in a greater likelihood of classical conditioning occurring in high Neuroticism scorers (Eysenck and Eysenck, 1985).

There is considerable evidence that scores on the Neuroticism scale (N scale) are linked to anxiety levels. A test of the importance of this factor is provided by a study which compared the Neuroticism scores of regular attenders with those of patients who had avoided the dentist for long periods. The avoidant group consisted of patients who volunteered for a treatment programme designed to reduce dental anxiety. The comparison group was made up of patients who had identified themselves as regular attenders and whose dentists considered them to be cooperative and relatively fearless.

Those in the avoidant group gave significantly higher scores on the Neuroticism scale than the regular attenders. Because Neuroticism seems to be linked with physiological characteristics, these results suggest that anxiety can sometimes be explained by reference to innate mechanisms. An interesting finding was that part of the effect appeared to be due to the low-fear group giving lower Neuroticism scores than the general population, so that the difference was not due wholly to the elevated scores of the avoidant group (Klepac et al., 1982).

Childhood characteristics: temperament

Children vary in many ways. Some are more easily distracted from tasks than others, some are predominately happy while others are more moody, and so on. While experiences are, of course, important in affecting such characteristics, there is now good evidence that they are partly genetically determined. They can emerge at a young age and persist over many years. Two important temperamental characteristics are known as *approach–withdrawal* and *adaptability*. A child who responds positively to a new situation (by smiling and moving towards it) can be contrasted with a child who responds negatively (by fussing and pulling away). Furthermore, some children adapt quickly to new situations while others take much longer.

A number of studies (Williams et al., 1985; Lochary et al., 1993; Radis et al., 1994) have showed the relevance of these characteristics to dentistry. Children referred to hospital for their anxiety have been found to be more likely to withdraw from novel situations in general and to have difficulty in adapting to change. This suggests that such children will have more problems with entering the dental office, even in the absence of any negative experience, and will require a more gradual introduction.

Taken together, the work on childhood characteristics and Neuroticism would suggest that some people with high levels of dental anxiety also have a number of other anxieties and concerns. This is an important issue, since it bears upon the possibility that dental anxiety and phobia can be indicative of more general psychological or psychiatric difficulties, rather than being a specific difficulty. There is now growing evidence that this is often, but not always, the case. A study by Roy-Bryne et al. (1994) indicated that in a sample of phobic patients, 40% could be assigned another concurrent psychiatric diagnosis, such as panic disorder.

Summary

Anxiety can be considered in a number of ways. Extraction, drilling and injection are the most anxiety-provoking features for most dental patients. There are important individual differences in how people react to these procedures, however, and several questionnaires have been developed to measure the amount of subjective anxiety a patient feels. The STAI distinguishes between trait anxiety (a long-term discomfort) and state anxiety (which depends on the particular situation). There are several questionnaires designed specifically for dental patients, such as the DAS.

Anxiety can be manifested in several ways. Physiological arousal may occur, signalled by a high pulse rate or sweating. Behaviourally, children might show their anxiety by refusing to cooperate when in the dental chair, while adults may be more likely to miss appointments or refuse to attend altogether. Scores of subjective, physiological and behavioural variables do not always agree, indicating that these components may operate independently from each other.

Patients often report that their anxiety stems from a fear of pain, and this is consistent with a classical conditioning explanation. But this does not provide a complete explanation since many people who expect pain or have had negative experiences in the past do not seem anxious. Some patients may be anxious because they are uncertain about what they will experience, while others may be particularly vulnerable to learning anxiety responses. It could be useful to consider all of these influences when attempting to alleviate anxiety, the topic of the next chapter.

Practice implications

- Different people show and experience anxiety in different ways, so it is not always possible to tell how anxious a patient might be. Anxiety levels might be higher in the waiting room, so a receptionist's judgement might be useful.
- Anxiety can 'run in families', so that a new child patient might experience a level of anxiety similar to that of the parent.
- Because the dental setting may be inherently anxiety provoking, the development of trust is crucial.
- A gradual introduction might be especially helpful for children who have trouble entering or adapting to new situations.

References

American Psychiatric Association (1995). *Diagnostic and Statistical Manual of Mental Disorders. DSM-IV.* Washington DC: American Psychiatric Association.

Arntz, A., van Eck, M. and Heijmans, M. (1990). Predictions of dental pain: the fear of any expected evil is worse than the evil itself. *Behav. Res. Ther.,* **28**, 29–41.

Bailey, P., Talbot, A. and Taylor, P. P. (1973). A comparison of maternal anxiety levels with anxiety levels manifested in the child dental patient. *J. Dent. Child.,* **40**, 25–32.

Berggren, U. (1993). Psychosocial effects associated with dental fear in adult dental patients with avoidance behaviours. *Psychol. Health,* **8**, 185–196.

Bernstein, D., Kleinknecht, R. and Alexander, L. (1979). Antecedents of dental fear. *J. Public Health Dent.,* **39**, 113–124.

Brown, D., Wright, F. and McMurray, N. (1986). Psychological and behavioural factors associated with dental anxiety in children. *J. Behav. Med.,* **9**, 213–217.

Corah, N. (1969). Development of a dental anxiety scale. *J. Dent. Res.,* **48**, 596.

Corah, N., Gale, E. and Illig, S. (1978). Assessment of a dental anxiety scale. *J. Am. Dent. Assoc.,* **97**, 816–819.

Corkey, B. and Freeman, R. (1994). Predictors of dental anxiety in six-year-old children: findings from a pilot study. *J. Dent. Child.,* **61**, 267–271.

Curson, I. and Coplans, M. (1970). The need for sedation in conservative dentistry. *Br. Dent. J.,* **125**, 18–22.

Davey, G. (1989). Dental phobias and anxieties: evidence for conditioning processes in the acquisition and modulation of a learned fear. *Behav Res. Ther.,* **27**, 51–58.

de Jongh A. and Stouthard M. (1993) Anxiety about dental hygienist treatment. *Community Dent. Oral Epidemiol.,* **21**, 91–95.

de Jongh, A., Muris, P., ter Horst, G., Van-Zuuren, F. and De Wit, C. (1994). Cognitive correlates of dental anxiety. *J. Dent. Res.*, **73**, 561–566.

de Jongh, A., Muris, N., Schoenmakers, N., et al. (1995). Negative cognitions of dental phobics: reliability and validity of the dental cognitions questionnaire. *Behav. Res. Ther.*, **33**, 507–515.

de Silva, P. (1988). Phobias and preparedness: replication and extension. *Behav. Res. Ther.*, **26**, 97–98.

Epstein, S. and Roupenian, A. (1970). Heart rate and skin conductance during experimentally induced anxiety. The effect of uncertainty about receiving a noxious stimulus. *J. Pers. Soc. Psychol.*, **16**, 20–28.

Eysenck, H. and Eysenck, S. (1985). *Personality and Individual Differences*. Springfield: Thomas.

Fogione, A. and Clarke, R. (1974). Comments on an empirical study of the causes of dental fears. *J. Dent. Res.*, **53**, 496.

Frankl, S., Shiere, F. and Fogels, H. (1962). Should the parent remain with the child in the dental operatory? *J. Dent. Child.*, **29**, 150–163.

Gale, E. (1972). Fears of the dental situation. *J. Dent. Res.*, **51**, 964–966.

Gale, E. and Ayer, W. (1969). Treatment of dental phobias. *J. Am. Dent. Assoc.*, **73**, 1304–1307.

Hakeberg, M., Berggren, U. and Carlsson, S. (1992). Prevalence of dental anxiety in an adult population in a major urban area in Sweden. *Community Dent. Oral Epidemiol.*, **20**, 97–101.

Hall, N. and Edmondson, H. (1983). The aetiology and psychology of dental fear. *Br. Dent. J.*, **154**, 247–252.

Humphris, G., Morrison, T. and Lindsay, S. (1995). The modified dental anxiety scale: validation and United Kingdom norms. *Community Dent. Oral Epidemiol.*, **12**, 143–150.

Jackson, E. (1978). Patients' perceptions of dentistry. In *Advances in Behavioural Research in Dentistry*. (P. Weinstein, ed.) Department of Community Dentistry, University of Washington.

Johnson, R. and Baldwin, D. (1968). Relationship of maternal anxiety to the behaviour of young children undergoing dental extraction. *J. Dent. Res.*, **47**, 801–805.

Kagan, J. and Havemann, E. (1976). *Psychology. An Introduction*. New York: Harcourt Brace Jovanovich.

Kent, G., Rubin, G., Getz, T. and Humphris, G. (1996). The development of a scale to measure the social and psychological effects of severe dental anxiety. *Community Dent. Oral Epidemiol.* **24**, 394–397.

Kleinknecht, R. and Bernstein, D. (1978). The assessment of dental fear. *Behav. Ther.*, **9**, 626–634.

Kleinknecht, R., Klepac, R. and Alexander, L. (1973). Origins and characteristics of fear of dentistry. *J. Am. Dent. Assoc.*, **86**, 842–848.

Klepac, R., Dowling, J. and Hauge, G. (1982). Characteristics of clients seeking therapy for the reduction of dental avoidance: reactions to pain. *J. Behav. Ther. Exp. Psychiatry*, **13**, 293–300.

Klingberg, G., Berggren, U. and Noren, J. (1993). Dental fear in an urban Swedish child population: prevalence and concomitant factors. *Community Dent. Health*, **11**, 208–214.

Klorman, R., Michael, R., Hilpert, P., et al. (1979). A further assessment of predictors of the child's behaviour in dental treatment. *J. Dent. Res.*, **58**, 2338–2343.

Koenigsberg, S. and Johnson, R. (1972). Child behaviour during sequential dental visits. *J. Am. Dent. Assoc.*, **85**, 128–132.

Lautch, H. (1971). Dental phobia. *Br. J. Psychiatry*, **119**, 151–158.

Lochary, M., Wilson, S., Griffen, A. and Coury, D. (1993). Temperament as a predictor of behavior for conscious sedation. *Ped. Dent.*, **15**, 348–352.

Locker, D., Shapiro, D. and Liddell, A. (1996). Who is dentrally anxious? Concordance between measures of dental anxiety. *Community Dent. Oral Epidemiol.*, **24**, 346–350.

Ludwick, W., Schnoebelen, E. O. and Knoedler, D. J. (1964). *Greater Utilization of Dental Technicians. II. Report of Clinical Tests.* Mimeograph. Great Lakes: RUS Naval Training Center, Dental Research Facility.

Melamed, B., Weinstein, D., Hawes, R., et al. (1975). Reduction of fear-related dental management using filmed modeling. *J. Am. Dent. Assoc.*, **90**, 822–826.

Milgrom, P., Weinstein, P. and Getz, T. (1995). *Treating Fearful Dental Patients: A Patient Management Handbook*, 2nd edn. Seattle: University of Washington.

Moore, R., Brodsgaard, I. and Birn, H. (1991). Manifestations, acquisition and diagnostic categories of dental fear in a self-referred population. *Behav. Res. Ther.*, **29**, 51–60.

Moore, R., Kirkegaard, E., Brodsgaard, I. and Scheutz, F. (1993). Prevalence and characteristics of dental anxiety in Danish adults. *Community Dent. Oral Epidemiol.*, **21**, 292–296.

Murray, P., Liddell, A. and Donohue, J. (1989). A longitudinal study of the contribution of dental experience to dental anxiety in children between 9 and 12 years of age. *J. Behav. Med.*, **12**, 309–320.

Naitkin, E. and Guild, R. (1967). Evaluation of pre-clinical performance. *J. Dent. Educ.*, **31**, 152–161.

Neverlien, P. (1994). Dental anxiety, optimism–pessimism, and dental experience from childhood to adolescence. *Community Dent. Oral Epidemiol.*, **22**, 263–268.

Radis, F., Wilson, S., Griffen, A. and Coury, D. (1994). Temperament as a predictor of behavior during initial dental examination in children. *Ped. Dent.*, **16**, 121–127.

Rosenberg, H. and Katcher, A. (1976). Heart rate and physical activity of children during dental treatment. *J. Dent. Res.*, **55**, 648–651.

Roy-Bryne, P., Milgrom, P., Khoon-Mei, T., et al. (1994). Psychopathology and psychiatric diagnosis in subjects with dental phobia. *J. Anxiety Disorders*, **8**, 19–31.

Schuurs, A. and Hoogstraten, J. (1993). Appraisal of dental anxiety and fear questionnaires: a review. *Community Dent. Oral Epidemiol.*, **21**, 329–339.

Segal, H. (1986). Categories of emergency patient. *Gen. Dent.*, **34**, 37–42.

Semet, O. (1974). Emotional and medical factors in child dental anxiety. *J. Child Psychol. Psychiatry*, **15**, 313–321.

Shaw, O. (1975). Dental anxiety in children. *Br. Dent. J.*, **139**, 134–139.

Shoben, E. and Borland, L. (1954). An empirical study of the aetiology of dental fears. *J. Clin. Psychol.*, **10**, 171–174.

Simpson, W. J., Ruzicka, R. L. and Thomas, H. R. (1974). Physiologic responses to initial dental experience. *J. Dent. Child.*, **41**, 465–470.

Speilberger, C., Gorsuch, R. and Lushene, R. (1983). *STAI Manual for the State–Trait Inventory.* Palo Alto: Consulting Psychologists Press.

Stewart, J., Marcus, M., Christenson, P. and Lin, W. (1994). Comprehensive treatment among dental school patients with high and low dental anxiety. *J. Dent. Educ.*, **58**, 697–700.

Stouthard, M. and Hoogstraten, J. (1990). Dental anxiety: a comparison of dentate and edentulous subjects. *Community Dent. Oral Epidemiol.*, **18**, 267–268.

ter Horst, G. and de Wit, C. (1993). Review of behavioural research in dentistry 1987–1992: Dental anxiety, dentist–patient relationship, compliance and dental attendance. *Int. Dent. J.*, **43**, 265–278.

Todd, J. E. and Walker, A. (1980). *Adult Dental Health in England and Wales.* London:

HMSO.

Todd, J. E., Walker, A. and Dodd, P. (1982). *Adult Dental Health, United Kingdom.* London: HMSO.

Tullman, G., Tullman, M., Rogers, B., et al. (1979). Anxiety in dental patients: a study of three phases of state anxiety in three treatment groups. *Psychol. Rep.,* **45**, 407–412.

Venham, L. (1979). The effect of mother's presence on child's response to dental treatment. *J. Dent. Child.,* **46**, 219–225.

Wardle, J. (1982a). Fear of dentistry. *Br. J. Med. Psychol.,* **55**, 119–126.

Wardle, J. (1982b). *Management of Dental Pain.* Paper presented at the British Psychological Society Annual Conference, York.

Watson, J. and Raynor, R. (1920). Conditioned emotional reactions. *J. Exp. Psychol.,* **3**, 1–14.

Williams, J. M. G., Murray, J., Lund, C., Harkiss, B. and de Franco, A. (1985). Anxiety in the child dental clinic. *J. Child Psychol. Psychiatry,* **26**, 305–310.

Chapter 6

Alleviating anxiety

In the previous chapter, we considered research on two aspects of anxiety. The first was a discussion of the four components – the situation, subjective reports, physiological arousal and behaviour – which have proved useful in understanding the nature of anxiety. In the second part of Chapter 5, we also considered the causes of anxiety. Patients' concerns are often focused on pain, but the dentist's personality, the uncertainty of dental care, previous learning experiences and biological predisposition can be important influences on these worries. There are many advantages in helping patients with their anxiety. Not only might it improve the quality of dentists' professional lives, but there is evidence that treatment can have positive effects on a variety of psychosocial measures such as patients' days off work (Hakeberg and Berggren, 1992).

Preventing anxiety

Many clues about how to alleviate anxiety in dental patients can be gained from the research outlined in the previous chapter. Perhaps the best method is good prevention. Since negative experiences can sometimes lead to future anxiety, a reduction in the need for extractions and fillings would be a priority. Here the benefits of fluoridation of public water supplies and the importance of involving parents in their children's diet and oral hygiene habits become clear. If dental care is given on a regular basis and is restricted to examination and cleaning, then early traumatic experiences could be eliminated to a large extent.

For children, the most important preventive measure is the provision of an environment in which they feel safe and trusting. This cannot be achieved immediately. It is important to take each individual child's needs into account by listening to and reacting to his or her communications. Many dentists argue that the actual accomplishment of treatment is always secondary to the establishment of trust when a new patient enters the office.

Although some people are frightened of injections, it is probable that the use of local anaesthetics has made a significant contribution to the reduction of dental anxiety among the public. Many older patients report that although they were frightened of dentistry when younger, repeated visits over their lifetime have relieved their anxiety. This can be explained through extinction: patients who had been very anxious about dental care because it was associated with pain in the past may have come to learn that this association is no longer present after a series of pain-free visits. However, it should be noted that local anaesthetics sometimes fail, and anxious patients are more likely to report a history of failure to get numb (Kaufman et al., 1984).

Persistent anxiety

Where anxiety has developed and persists, however, several kinds of procedure might be followed. For those patients who feel pain despite the use of local anaesthetics, psychological methods have been developed to lessen this discomfort, as discussed in the next chapter. Other patients who have found the behaviour and attitudes of their dentist worrying may be helped if the dentist can relieve these apprehensions. One patient might be anxious because of uncertainty about what procedures a treatment may involve, while another might be concerned lest the dentist criticizes oral hygiene habits.

Pharmacological approaches

Pharmacological methods of anxiety relief provide another possibility. A general anaesthetic can be used in extreme cases but is inappropriate for most cases of anxiety. Many dentists are reluctant to use it, partly because of the dangers involved and partly because it does not help the patient to come to terms with anxiety and learn how to cope with it.

An alternative pharmacological method is relative analgesia, which involves the inhalation of a mixture of nitrous oxide and oxygen. Roberts et al. (1979) studied the effects of relative analgesia on 65 children between four and 17 years of age, all of whom had shown uncooperative behaviour in the dental chair previously. When the children arrived for their appointments, their anxiety was judged according to the following categories: uncontrollable; extremely nervous; very nervous; slightly nervous; or not nervous. The amount of anxiety shown by the children as they arrived for their three visits is shown in Figure 6.1. At the beginning of the first visit over 70% of the children were rated as being extremely or very nervous, but by the beginning of the third visit only 25% of the remaining children (some had completed treatment) were so judged. Cooperation improved in over 90% of the patients during this time and there was no indication of any adverse physiological effects. A follow-up of these children indicated that most were able to accept treatment at a later date without nitrous oxide sedation. It seems that success at the first session is very important for a child's ability to cope in later sessions (Veerkamp et al., 1993). Thus it would seem that this technique has some rehabilitative properties.

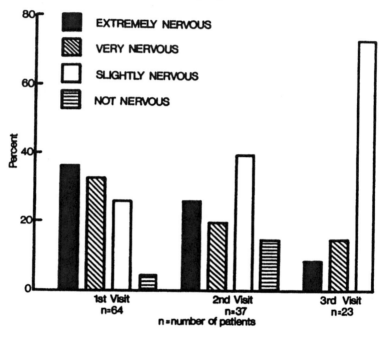

Figure 6.1. Assessment of anxiety at the beginning of each visit for children given relative analgesia. From Roberts et al. (1979), with permission.

Hall and Edmondson (1983) reported that intravenous diazepam, a tranquillizer, can have significant long-term effects on patients' fears. Of 70 phobic patients, 65 completed the initial course of treatment (for two treatment was abandoned and three were rendered edentulous). Of the 49 patients who could be traced five years later, only three had no further dental care since the initial treatment. Thirty were receiving treatment with local anaesthesia only, while 16 still required intravenous sedation. Recently, there has been much interest in the use of midazolam as a sedative, but there is great variation in its effectiveness (Ellis, 1996).

These pharmacological approaches can be helpful, but the purpose of this chapter is to discuss psychological methods of alleviating anxiety. In the longer term they can be of greater benefit (Berggren and Linde, 1984). This is, of course, an advantage to the dentist as well, in that the time invested in helping anxious patients may be rewarded by fewer disruptions to scheduling and more satisfying relationships. A variety of techniques are discussed below. Hypnosis, which is becoming increasingly popular amongst dentists, is covered in the next chapter on pain, but it can also be effective in reducing anxiety (Shaw and Niven, 1996).

Some basic principles

Four central ideas underlie all of the treatments discussed in this chapter. They are:

1. The methods provide patients with increasing degrees of experience with the dental situation.
2. Exposure to the situation is increased gradually, so that a patient's coping strategies are not overwhelmed.
3. The aim is to help a patient manage his or her anxiety by increasing coping strategies, especially by increasing a sense of control or by changing perceptions of the dental setting.
4. Anxious patients are often ashamed of their difficulties and may be concerned about being judged negatively. Whatever the approach used, it is important to be accepting and non-evaluative.

Modelling

Modelling is based on the idea that people learn much about their environment from observing the consequences of others' behaviour. In our culture, where dentistry is considered painful and something to be avoided, children in particular may come to fear a visit to the dentist because they have heard about other people's negative experiences. Conversely, modelling could be used to alleviate anxiety. If a patient could be shown that it is possible to visit the dentist, have treatment and then leave without undue distress, anxiety might be reduced. Modelling could also be effective through the reduction of uncertainty. While observing someone undergo an examination or treatment, the patient would be gaining information about the kinds of equipment he or she will encounter and would learn which kinds of behaviour are acceptable.

Experiments on modelling

Melamed et al. (1975) tested the effect of modelling for children aged 5–9, most of whom had little direct experience of dentistry. During the experiment, all were seen by the dentist three times: a radiograph was taken on the first visit, an examination was given on the second and restorations were given on the third. Just before this last visit, one-half of the patients were shown a film of a four-year-old child undergoing a restoration. The child on the film was praised by the dentist for his cooperative behaviour and was rewarded with a small toy at the end of the session. The remaining patients formed the control group, being asked to draw pictures for the same time interval as the film took to view.

Melamed et al. made several measures of anxiety during all three visits, including the amount and frequency of disruptive behaviour (e.g. crying, kicking, refusing to open the mouth). As shown in Figure 6.2, the differences between the groups are insignificant at the first and second visits, but a large difference was found on the third (treatment) visit. Those children who viewed the film continued to show a moderately low level of disruption despite the increased demands placed upon them. By contrast, the disruption shown by the control group children increased considerably.

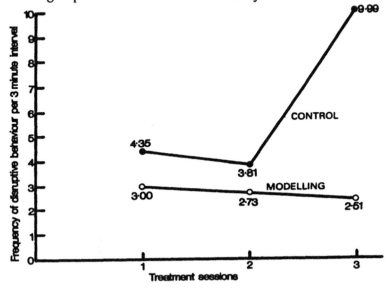

Figure 6.2. Frequency of disruptive behaviour in the modelled and control groups when (1) radiographs were taken, (2) the children's teeth were examined, and (3) restorations were placed. From Melamed et al. (1975), with permission.

Using films

Later research (e.g. Melamed et al., 1978) has indicated that care should be taken when developing and using such films. There is some evidence that for children with no prior experience of visiting the dentist, showing a film demonstrating procedures without a model could have a sensitizing effect, in that these children can become more disruptive. One important factor concerns the effects of including a model in the films as opposed to having the dentist simply describe what he or she was doing. Children who view films with a model report fewer fears and show less disruptive behaviour than children who view films that demonstrate only equipment.

There are several other points. The model should show cooperation during treatment and be praised for this behaviour. The age of the model is significant, in that the best results are gained when the model is close in age to the target children. The model should also be shown leaving the surgery in much the same way as he or she arrived, thus indicating that the treatment does not have any lasting adverse effects. While not all studies show such positive results, it is important that the dentist is portrayed as a caring individual who is concerned about the patient.

Using live models

It is not necessary to use films, however. Stokes and Kennedy (1980) describe how they arranged for some very disruptive children to arrive 10–15 minutes before their treatment was due to begin. The children were invited to observe the previous child being treated, who was praised and rewarded for being cooperative. Over four visits, the amount of disruptive behaviour shown by the children decreased by over two-thirds.

Family members can also be used if they have a low level of anxiety. In a case report, Klesges and Malott (1984) asked the mother of a four-year-old dentally phobic girl to model coping behaviour, while Ghose et al. (1969) used siblings. In the latter study, both siblings entered the surgery together and the younger child watched while the older was examined and treated. Interestingly, these effects held only for children aged four years – no differences were found for those aged three and five years – and were strongest when the sibling relationship was 'good' rather than 'fair' or 'poor'.

Participant modelling

Participant modelling requires more patient involvement. Here, patients not only see a model undergo treatment but also go through the procedures themselves immediately afterwards. In the first instance this can be simulated, the patient graduating to actual treatment later on. For example, Bernstein and Kleinknecht (1982) arranged for fearful patients to observe a model demonstrating the various steps needed in order to obtain professional care: telephoning a dentist, arriving at the surgery, receiving an oral examination, and so on. Then the patients repeated each step themselves, only moving on to the next one when they felt comfortable. As each step was completed, they were praised for their progress. This approach seemed very useful, in that 87.5% of the patients, all of whom had avoided the dentist for up to 10 years, subsequently kept an appointment for treatment.

Reducing uncertainty

While modelling is an effective approach for reducing anxiety, it seems likely that at least some of the effect is due to the reduction of uncertainty and the reassurance given by a friendly and caring dentist. Since uncertainty raises anxiety, providing patients with information about their treatment would be expected to reduce it. Sometimes even small points of information, such as the expected length of the appointment, can be very helpful.

Many people will not understand the reason for dental procedures or the use of dental instruments. This is particularly true for children. For example, Eiser et al. (1983) found that more than half of the six-year-olds they questioned did not know what an injection was. Children may also have misconceptions about dentistry: young children in particular may see the experience of discomfort as a punishment for past misbehaviour.

Tell Show Do

This is one method which has achieved much popularity as a way of introducing children to dental equipment and procedures. The Tell phase involves an age-appropriate explanation of the procedures and the reasons for their use. The Show phase is used to demonstrate a procedure, up to the point where the instrument is actually used. A cotton swab, rather than the needle, might be used to indicate the position of an anaesthetic injection. In a matter-of-fact way and with a minimum of delay, the Do phase is initiated. Throughout, the dentist seeks to relax the child and praise appropriate and cooperative behaviour. Unfortunately, in what seems to be the only experiment to have evaluated this approach (Howitt and Stricker, 1965), there was no evidence that it was effective for highly anxious children. It may be more useful for children with lower levels of anxiety.

Preparatory information

Other methods, which have involved preparing children and their parents for a first visit, have had some success. For example, Rosengarten (1961) posted preparatory information to some parents who were due to bring their children to the dentist for the first time. This included a short booklet to be read to the children. On their first visit, no treatment or examination was given, but instead the children were simply introduced to the office, the dentist and the hygienist. This preparation resulted in more cooperation being shown than for children not given the introduction, at least for those aged 3–4 years.

It is not clear whether it was the visit or the booklet which was important for these children. In studies where parents have been given a pre-appointment letter alone (such as that shown in Table 6.1), the mothers have found them helpful (Wright et al., 1973) and there has been a reduced number of broken appointments (Hawley et al., 1974). However, there has been little effect on the actual behaviour of the children.

Table 6.1. An example of a letter that could be sent to parents before their child's first dental visit

---

Your child's first dental visit

Dear

I am writing to you because I am pleased with the interest you are showing in your child's dental health by making an appointment for a dental examination. Children who have their first dental appointment when they are very young are likely to have a favourable outlook toward dental care throughout life.

At our first appointment, we will examine your child's teeth and gums and take any necessary X-rays. For most children, this proves to be an interesting and even happy occasion.

All of the people on our staff enjoy children and know how to work with them. Parents play a most important role in getting children started with a good attitude toward dental care, and your cooperation is much appreciated. One of the useful things you can do is to be completely natural and easy-going when you tell your child about the appointment with the dentist. This approach will enable him/her to view it primarily as an opportunity to meet some new people who are interested in him/her and want him/her to stay healthy.

Good general health depends in large part upon the development of good habits, such as sensible eating and sleeping routines, exercise, recreation and the like. Dental health also depends upon good habits, including tooth brushing, regular visits to the dentist and avoidance of excessive amounts of sweets. We will have a chance to discuss these points further during your child's appointment.

Best wishes, and I look forward to seeing you.

From Wright et al. (1973), with permission.

Preparation for extractions

When pre-visit preparation is given, it may be important to provide children with some time in order to accommodate themselves to dental procedures. Baldwin and Barnes (1966) compared the reactions of children who had extractions with those whose treatment was more routine. Usually, children were told about an extraction 4–7 days before it was due to occur. Perhaps this was the cause of their distress: they had up to a week to worry about the extraction, and time to become more and more concerned. Such a view would be consistent with the idea that children should not be told about treatment lest they worry about it.

In order to test the importance of a waiting period, Baldwin and Barnes arranged for a group of children to be given their extractions on the same day that they were informed about them. There were some interesting interview data from the children and their parents. Every one of the children said that they would prefer to be warned in advance about dental extractions, expressed as a need to 'think about it', or 'get ready for it'. They said they wanted this time 'to get used to the idea' or 'to ask my friends about it'. Two of the children from the no-waiting group spontaneously remarked that they could never again be sure that when they went to the dentist he might not suddenly decide to take out a tooth. It seemed that the waiting period was, indeed, helpful.

In contrast, less than 50% of the parents thought their children should be told ahead of time. Some parents suggested that 'he'll just get scared' or 'why make him worry, there's enough time for that later in life'. Typical comments of those parents who felt that a waiting period was helpful were 'he's better off if he has time to think about it' and 'I always tell him what will happen'. Baldwin and Barnes suggested that one reason why children are pushed into surgery quickly is that the parents cannot cope with their own anxieties about it, as indicated by those who expressed such comments as 'I'm glad I'm not him today, I'm more nervous than he is'.

Amount of information given to patients

This idea of preparing patients for treatment by explaining what is going to happen to them well in advance is a most important one and will be discussed further in the next chapter on pain. However, it is also possible to provide too much information for children on their first visit. It would be a mistake to work on the principle that if a little information is good, then more would be better.

Herbertt and Innes (1979) varied the amount of information they gave to their patients about treatment procedures. Some children received little treatment information, only being given a short lesson in dental health. Additional information was added for other groups until it was very detailed and thorough. The relationship between anxiety and information was curvilinear: too much or too little treatment information resulted in higher anxiety. When introducing a child to dentistry, it seems important that a gradual approach be used: one that allows a child to assimilate the new environment slowly.

Personality
Another reason why it is important to be careful not to provide too much information about treatment involves personality differences. It seems that the recovery of some people is actually hindered by giving them more information than they want (Auerbach and Kilman, 1977). Unwanted information can override patients' ways of coping, making it more difficult for them.

The personality characteristic of locus of control is relevant here. Some people tend to believe that what happens to them is mainly a result of chance or fate and there is little they can do to change things. Such people are said to have an 'external' locus of control. Other people, by contrast, tend to believe that events are largely under their own control and that they can effect outcomes, termed an 'internal' locus of control. Auerbach et al. (1976) gave a questionnaire designed to measure locus of control to patients when they arrived at a dental clinic to have an extraction. They then showed two types of film. Some patients were shown a film containing general information: it described the clinic and some of the equipment they would encounter. Other patients were given much more specific information: they were told why extractions were sometimes necessary, a description of how the anaesthetic was given, the method of extraction was demonstrated and some ways to alleviate pain afterwards were suggested.

In order to measure anxiety, the oral surgeons rated how the patients reacted to the treatment. This judgement was based on how they responded to the anaesthetic, their degree of cooperation and the amount of pain they reported. The scores of these various ratings were combined to give a total adjustment score, as shown in Figure 6.3. The 'internal' patients showed better adjustment during the extraction if they viewed the specific information film, while this was not the case for the 'external' patients. For them, there was a tendency to show poorer adjustment.

Thus, with both adults and children, it is important to be sensitive to individual requirements. It is important for the dentist to be open

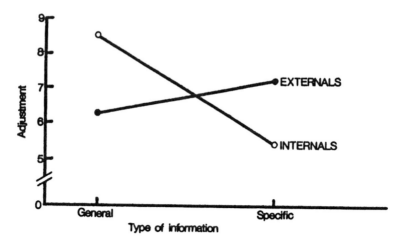

Figure 6.3. Adjustment shown by patients with external and internal locus of control when given either specific or general information about an extraction. A higher score represented poorer adjustment. Adapted from Auerbach et al. (1976), with permission.

to the type and amount of information that individual patients need. In many instances it is not what dentists tell patients that is important, but rather what dentists allow patients to tell them.

Enhancing control

One reason why uncertainty may be related to anxiety is that when people have little idea of what is going to happen to them, they have little opportunity to alter their own or the dentist's behaviour. Weinstein and Nathan (1988) argue that providing children with a sense of control is particularly important because of their feelings of vulnerability. They suggest that a sense of control can be enhanced by giving a multitude of small choices, such as asking children which side of the chair they would like to get up, whether they would like their top or bottom teeth cleaned first, offering a rest from procedures, and so on.

Stop signals

The idea that having control can reduce anxiety can be tested directly by giving patients a means of signalling their discomfort to the dentist. Corah (1973) explored this idea with children aged 6–11 years. One group of children was given routine dental care. The other group was told that they could change their dentist's behaviour by pushing one of two buttons. When one button was pressed, a green light would shine in front of the dentist. This could be used to indicate that the procedure was bothering the patient but not so much that he wanted the dentist to stop working. Another button lit a red light and sounded a buzzer: this was to be used when the children wanted the dentist to stop for a short while until they felt more comfortable. On a galvanic skin response measure, the group of children given the buttons to push showed lower anxiety to highly stressful procedures (e.g. injection, drilling) but not to low-stress ones (e.g. placing amalgam).

A more practical approach than using buttons is to ask patients to indicate that they want the dentist to stop or pause by raising an arm or hand. This type of stop signal is very widely used and is effective in reducing pain (Thrash et al., 1982) as well as anxiety. It might be particularly helpful for new patients to know that their dentist recommends stop signals. Jackson and Lindsay (1995) demonstrated that a short leaflet which informed the patients that they could stop their dentist during treatment was effective in reducing the anxiety they were feeling just before their appointment.

Emotional support

While the anxiety associated with uncertainty can be reduced by providing information, dentists are also providing emotional support when they take the time to explain the nature of procedures and treatment. There is the implicit message that the dentist is aware of the anxieties inherent in the situation and is attempting to reduce them. This provides some security and trust.

A study on children who were about to have a minor operation (Fassler, 1980) illustrates this clearly. One group of children was given extensive preparation for their hospitalization. They were read a story about a child going to the hospital and given a set of hospital toys to play with which could be used to depict hospital scenes. The children were also encouraged to express any fears and doubts about their operation and any misconceptions were corrected. This intervention thus involved both factual information and emotional reassurance — how important was the emotional support? In order to look at this, another intervention was included in the study. A second group of children was given emotional support but no direct information. They, too, heard a story, were given toys and were engaged in conversation, but the conversation centred around school and friends rather than hospitalization, and the toys and story did not

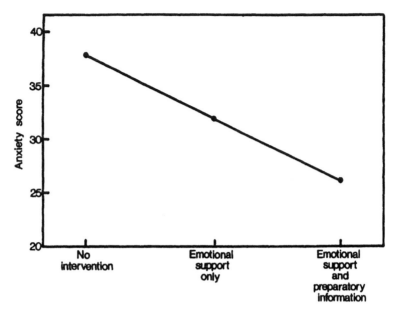

Figure 6.4. Anxiety scores for hospitalized children who had received no intervention, received emotional support, or received both emotional support and preparatory information. From Fassler (1980), with permission.

concern hospitals. The third group of children were given no additional emotional support or preparatory information.

All the children were then asked about their present feelings. The results for the three conditions are shown in Figure 6.4: those given emotional support plus information reported the lowest anxiety, followed by those given emotional support alone, while the no-intervention group showed the highest anxiety levels. Thus, emotional support alone had a beneficial effect on anxiety and this was further enhanced by giving preparatory information.

While few dentists will be able to spend so much time with their child patients, it is useful to recall the results of a study mentioned in the previous chapter. There, university students were asked to write an essay describing their visits to the dentist as children, including those events which influenced their present attitudes. The personality of the dentist was significant for the students, with many of them recalling their dentist as being either 'cold' and 'uncaring' or 'warm' and 'friendly'. Even in these relatively brief encounters, the emotional support given by their dentists had a lasting effect on their feelings.

Parents in the surgery

It could be argued that the child's family is in the best position to offer emotional support, and this raises the important question of whether a child's parents or siblings should be allowed in the surgery during treatment. There is no conclusive evidence concerning the effects of a parent's presence in the dental surgery. The argument against letting a parent attend is that the child is more likely to 'play-up', but there is, at least, no evidence that disruption is more likely when a parent is present in the surgery (Fenlon et al., 1993). In some respects this might be considered an ethical rather than purely an empirical problem: does the dentist have the right to bar a parent who wishes to be present?

It may be that the absence of any effect in the studies in this area is due to the standard experimental procedure of randomly assigning parents and children to either present or absent conditions. As Venham (1979) puts it:

Some children clearly received strong support and security from the mother's presence. On several occasions, a child grasped the mother's hand. On the other hand, several mothers clearly exhibited behaviour that would tend to increase the child's anxiety. They openly expressed fear of the dentist and specific dental procedures in front of their children and asked to avoid seeing the procedure. These mothers moved nervously in their chairs, hid their eyes, displayed exaggerated facial signs of fear and emitted sounds associated with fear and anxiety, all in full view of their children. (p. 142).

A more sophisticated experimental procedure, where the anxiety of the parent is taken into account, may indicate that a parent's presence is helpful when he or she is calm, but unhelpful if he or she is anxious. In the latter case, the parent may require assistance, perhaps through some of the techniques discussed in this chapter. Incidentally, several dentists have noted that anxious parents sometimes send their children to a dentist first in order to gauge the dentist's abilities. By doing everything possible to relieve any anxiety the child might feel, the parent's fears might also be reduced, making it possible for them to seek treatment for themselves.

Relaxation

The idea behind the use of relaxation therapy is that anxiety is associated with certain kinds of physiological arousal: high heart rate, muscular tension and sweating. If a patient could be taught to control these signs of arousal, an important component of anxiety could be reduced.

Relaxation training

There are several methods for teaching relaxation. One approach uses biofeedback (e.g. Miller et al., 1978), but the problem with this is that it requires specialist equipment and is probably no more effective than alternative methods. The best-known and validated method is called progressive muscle relaxation. The patient is asked to sit in a comfortable reclining chair. The therapist then asks the patient to first tense and then relax the major muscle groups in the body. The procedure often starts with the toes and then works progressively through the ankles, calves, thighs, and so on. Slow and controlled breathing with the eyes shut is finally achieved. The exercise takes 15–25 minutes to complete and the patient would be asked to remain in this state for a further 10 minutes or so. For most people, this results in a general feeling of calm and relaxation, a feeling very different from that engendered by anxiety. After several training sessions, people can generally relax themselves fairly quickly without the presence of the therapist.

Lamb and Strand (1980) describe how they used this technique for dental patients who were scheduled for routine treatments. As they arrived, the patients were given the STAI anxiety questionnaire discussed in the previous chapter. One-half of the patients were then escorted to another room, seated in reclining chairs and asked to follow the instructions on a 14-minute audiotape which explained the muscle relaxation method. After this, the patients were again asked to fill out the anxiety questionnaire and were then accompanied to the dental chair. When the dental treatment was completed, the anxiety questionnaire was filled out twice more, once according to 'how you felt while you were in the dentist's chair' and finally according to 'how you feel right now'. The other half of the patients were not given the relaxation exercise but were asked to fill out the questionnaires at the same time points.

The results for the state anxiety measures are shown in Figure 6.5. For the relaxation group, the scores dropped after hearing the tape and did not rise significantly during the dental treatment. In contrast, the group not given relaxation training showed no decrease in anxiety until they had left the chair. This study shows that anxiety can be reduced with a minimum intervention by clinicians with only a small amount of formal training, and the intervention used in Lamb and Strand's study did not disrupt the patients' visit or the dentist's scheduling.

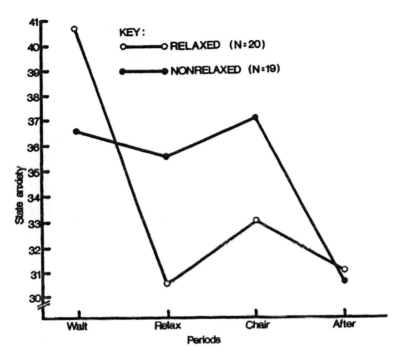

Figure 6.5. State anxiety scores for patients given and not given relaxation training. The anxiety of patients who heard a relaxation tape decreased before the treatment but the anxiety of the non-relaxed patients decreased only after treatment was completed. Adapted from Lamb and Strand (1980), with permission.

Systematic desensitization

The notion that patients could become less anxious about dentistry through repeated contacts is a familiar one: if an anxious patient finds that nothing distressing occurs on several occasions, the anxiety will eventually be reduced through extinction. However, this is rather haphazard and it may be years before anxiety eventually subsides, and it does not apply to patients who are so frightened of dentistry that they refuse even to enter the surgery. In systematic desensitization (SD), the process is formalized and it can be used for severely anxious patients.

The technique may be best described by outlining a case study (Gale and Ayer, 1969). The patient was a 32-year-old man who had a history of avoiding the dentist. He was taken to a dentist at the age of five or six, but tried to flee from the office. At eight years of age, he refused to have any dental work done. At 18 he had one filling and then refused to return. Later, after a toothache lasting three weeks, he finally went to a dentist who placed him under general anaesthetic. Several teeth were removed and several restorations completed. Over the next 12 years he suffered repeated toothaches but did not see a dentist.

During SD, the patient was seen by a therapist for nine sessions of about one hour each. At the first session, the patient's history was taken and relaxation therapy was begun. In the second session, further relaxation training was given and the patient was asked to list his fears about the restoration of his teeth. These fears were ordered in a hierarchy, as shown in Table 6.2. The least anxiety-provoking situation was thinking about going to the dentist, while the worst was receiving two injections, one on each side. Another list was made for extractions. In the third session, relaxation therapy was completed.

Table 6.2. Hierarchy of a patient's fears from least (1) to most (13) feared situation

1. Thinking about going to the dentist
2. Getting in your car to go to the dentist
3. Calling for an appointment with the dentist
4. Sitting in the waiting room of the dentist's office
5. Having the nurse tell you it's your turn
6. Getting in the dentist's chair
7. Seeing the dentist lay out the instruments, one of which is a probe
8. Having a probe held in front of you while you look at it
9. Having a probe placed on the side of a tooth
10. Having a probe placed in a cavity
11. Getting an injection in your gums on one side
12. Having your teeth drilled and worrying that the anaesthetic will wear off
13. Getting two injections, one on each side

From Gale and Ayer (1969), with permission.

The next six sessions were devoted to pairing the relaxation with the items in the hierarchy. In SD, this is done by asking the patient to relax as fully as possible. He is then requested to visualize the situations that he finds frightening, starting with the least frightening one. Whenever he feels anxious, the therapist instructs him to stop thinking about this situation and concentrate again on the relaxation. By pairing relaxation with the image, the situation begins to lose its anxiety-provoking properties. When the patient can visualize the least frightening situation without feeling anxious, he moves on to the next step of the hierarchy. This is repeated until he can think of the most frightening situation without becoming anxious. SD was very successful with this particular patient. Just before the ninth session, he made and kept an appointment with a dentist. Afterwards, all necessary dental treatment was completed and he found it 'relaxing'.

Cognitive approaches

While modelling is based on the idea that people can learn about the consequences of dental care from watching others, and the various types of relaxation training serve to inhibit physiological arousal, cognitive strategies operate on a different principle. Anxious dental patients often think about the worst possible consequences of dental care, for example, 'Any time now he will get the nerve and then it will really hurt'. For many anxious patients, it is not a question *if* they will experience pain, but *when*. Once these anxiety-laden thoughts come to mind, they heighten a patient's anxiety level, so that a vicious circle develops. If these kinds of anxiety-provoking thoughts can be prevented, then the anxiety itself could be reduced. The studies discussed under 'Reducing Uncertainty' earlier in the chapter could be included here since they also involve changing the way patients perceive the dental situation. In this section, two methods are outlined: distraction and cognitive modification.

Distraction

In this approach, the aim is to shift a patient's attention away from the dental setting and towards some other kind of situation. If a patient is thinking about something other than the dental work, he or she will be less likely to dwell on anxiety-provoking thoughts. It follows that the more a distractor 'captures' the patient's attention, the more effective it will be.

In one experiment (Corah et al., 1979a), adult patients who required at least two visits for restorations were studied. One group of patients was given no intervention, with their dental treatment proceeding as usual. A second group was asked to listen to a relaxation tape during treatment, through headphones. The tape asked the patients to relax their muscles as in progressive relaxation, except that the jaw muscles were excluded because this would interfere with the dentist's work. A third group of patients was assigned to a 'perceived control' group. They were told that they could ask the dentist to stop his work by pressing a button which would sound a buzzer. The dentist would then pause until the patient was more comfortable. The patients in the remaining group were given a way of distracting their attention from the treatment. A ping-pong video game, which they could play throughout the restoration, was mounted above their heads. This served to shift their attention away from the dentist's work.

The relaxation and distraction conditions were equally effective in reducing discomfort for anxious patients, and these two interventions were superior to the no-intervention condition. In the second study (Corah et al., 1979b), many of the same results were found, but there were some interesting sex differences. Distraction was generally more effective in reducing anxiety for men, while relaxation was better for women.

Distraction for children

There is some disagreement as to whether distraction is a helpful approach with children, with some studies finding that it is not effective. However, two reports indicate that the type of distractor and the way it is presented are crucial. Ingersoll et al. (1984a) encouraged children to view videotaped cartoons during treatment, but some children were told that the video would be switched off if they became uncooperative. For other children the video played regardless of their behaviour. The second condition had very little effect, their behaviour being similar to that of a control group who underwent treatment with no distractor available. However, the amount of disruptive behaviour was halved in the group who were told that the availability of the cartoons was contingent on their behaviour. In a later study (Ingersoll et al., 1984b), audiotaped stories were used: this was even more effective than the cartoons, perhaps because the children tended to close their eyes in order to concentrate on the stories, so the sights as well as the sounds of treatment were excluded. These studies indicate that (1) a distractor may be effective in changing behaviour only if there is some incentive and (2) some distractors are more effective than others.

Cognitive modification

While distraction aims to shift a patient's attention away from a distressing situation, the aim of cognitive modification is to focus attention on the positive aspects of treatment. Instead of dwelling on possible negative consequences, the patient is asked to concentrate on some positive possibilities, such as 'The dentist has never hurt me before and he won't do it now' or 'Once this appointment is finished, my teeth will be clean and healthy'.

Nelson (1981) illustrated this method in a case study of a young girl with a dental phobia. He first modelled coping self-statements (e.g. 'The dentist is really your friend') and then asked the girl to verbalize the statements herself. Several role-plays were used in which they practiced these statements. Over several appointments, anxiety decreased so that the girl was able to enter the dental setting with less anxiety and less disruptive behaviour.

Choosing between interventions

The evidence described thus far indicates that modelling, reducing uncertainty, providing emotional support, relaxation and the cognitive approaches are all effective in reducing anxiety. Most of these techniques have been tested on both normally and intensely anxious groups of patients with success. However, it should be noted that there is no one-to-one relationship between a reduction of measured anxiety and subsequent improvements in attendance (Schuurs et al., 1995). Nevertheless, with such a variety of effective methods available, an important question concerns when to use one technique in preference to another. If one kind of intervention could be shown to be superior to other kinds, then perhaps this would be the treatment of choice for most patients.

There are several studies in which some patients have received one type of intervention (e.g. practice in the use of distraction) or another (e.g. preparatory information). In general, about 60–80% of patients are helped regardless of the type of therapy, and in most studies, patients given some form of assistance are able to cope better than those given none. Patient variables may be important: there is some evidence that patients whose anxiety is limited to the dental setting, rather than being more generalized, are more likely to benefit (Berggren and Carlsson, 1985).

Common factors in therapies

Some psychologists have argued that this similarity of treatment effectiveness is due to most therapies having several features in common. The patient is given hope that his or her anxiety will be relieved, each type of therapy enhances coping methods and a sense of control, and the therapist is giving the patient time and attention which provides emotional support. These factors alone might be sufficient to reduce discomfort. Certainly, when the therapist is unfriendly or too business-like, the effectiveness of these interventions is much reduced. Another argument is that patients who have avoided the dentist in the past may want to test the effectiveness of their therapy by making and keeping a dental appointment. As one patient put it after completing therapy, 'I am very curious about how I will react when I go to the dentist' (Bernstein and Kleinknecht, 1982). Once they have made a visit, they may find that the experience is not as distressing as they anticipated it would be, e.g. 'I finally tried novocaine and when I realized that it didn't hurt to get a shot and that I couldn't feel anything while he was drilling, I felt stupid for being so afraid of getting my teeth filled' (Bernstein and Kleinknecht, 1982).

Matching therapy to patient

Other psychologists contend that this similarity in effectiveness is due to the way in which these experiments have been designed. Patients are usually assigned to various therapies on a random basis, so that individual differences in age, personality or previous experiences are equally distributed across conditions. Perhaps a patient whose anxiety is primarily behavioural in nature would receive most benefit from a participant modelling approach, while for another patient whose difficulty is more biologically based, a relaxation method would be better (Ning and Liddell, 1991). Patients tend to do better if they are given a treatment package that includes several interventions which target a range of behavioural, physiological and cognitive symptoms, rather than a single intervention (Gaudio and Nevid, 1991).

Patients' advice

Patients' own views are relevant. Many patients who are extremely nervous will expect or prefer some kind of pharmacological sedation (Lindsay et al., 1987), so a dentist who prefers a psychological approach will need to take this into consideration. When O'Shea et al. (1986) asked patients what they would do to relieve patients' anxiety if they were dentists, several methods were suggested, as shown in Table 6.3. There is a wide range of possibilities, so asking individual patients about their preference may help in making an appropriate choice (Rankin and Harris, 1984). Smith et al. (1987) asked a group of patients who had successfully completed a psychological intervention about which aspects helped them to tolerate treatment. The patients indicated that a number of factors were important, including the provision of information, the time taken to help them, perceptions of control, and the dentist understanding and listening to their concerns rather than treating them as 'silly'.

Table 6.3. Patients' advice on how to reduce anxiety

Provide an initial explanation of planned procedures
Provide an explanation and description of procedures as they are being performed
Instruct the patient to be calm
Warn that discomfort may occur at particular points in a procedure
Support the patient by showing concern and being reassuring
Help the patient redefine the experience away from pain by providing a new way of
    viewing the situation
Give the patient some control over procedures
Help the patient to cope, e.g. through breathing exercises
Provide a way of distracting the patient
Build trust
Show personal warmth
Start with minor things first

Clinical psychology

When a patient does not respond to such simple interventions as
relaxation training or a gradual introduction to the dental office (or if
the anxiety seems too intense even to attempt any intervention),
referral to a specialist may be appropriate. Clinical psychologists have
extensive training in the methods outlined in this chapter and can be
contacted either through a patient's general medical practitioner or
privately. Subsequently the psychologist may ask for the dentist's
cooperation in introducing the patient to the equipment or surgery.

Summary

Persistent anxiety in dental patients can be relieved in many ways.
Modelling provides a patient with an opportunity to see others
showing little distress while being treated and may be effective partly
because it removes some of the uncertainty involved in dental care.
Direct reduction of uncertainty is also effective: providing patients
with clear information about the kinds of equipment and procedures
they will encounter alleviates anxiety, particularly for those with an
'internal' locus of control. It is important to remember, however, that
it is possible to provide too much information for some patients,
particularly children, who may have difficulties in coping with the
equipment found in the surgery. Emotional support is very important
for this group of patients. Relaxation and systematic desensitization
operate by reducing the physiological arousal associated with
anxiety. Distraction can be another effective technique: by shifting
a patient's attention away from the dentist's work, that patient is less
likely to think about the possibility of pain.

Practice implications

- In order to prevent the development of anxiety, more attention should be given to the enhancement of trust than the completion of treatment for a new patient.
- Siblings, parents and other patients can be used as models.
- Although giving information can be helpful, avoid providing more detail than is needed.
- Many patients use distraction. They can be helped with this if provided with attention-capturing materials such as audiotaped stories.
- Patients have their own strategies for coping. These can be discovered and strengthened.
- Consult a clinical psychologist if necessary.

Suggested reading

A further overview of this area is given by Milgrom, P., Weinsten, P. and Getz, T. (1995). *Treating Fearful Dental Patients. A Patient Management Handbook.* Seattle: University of Washington.

References

Auerbach, S., Kendall, P., Cuttler, H. et al. (1976). Anxiety, locus of control, type of preparatory information and adjustment to dental surgery. *J. Consult. Clin. Psychol.,* **44**, 809–818.

Auerbach, S. and Kilman, P. (1977). Crisis intervention: a review of outcome research. *Psychol. Bull.,* **84**, 1189–1217.

Baldwin, D. and Barnes, M. (1966). The psychological value of a pre-surgical waiting period in the preparation of children for dental extraction. *Trans. Eur. Orthodont. Soc.,* 297–308.

Berggren, U. and Linde, A. (1984). Dental fear and avoidance: a comparison of two modes of treatment. *J. Dent. Res.,* **63**, 1223–1227.

Berggren, U. and Carlsson, S. (1985). Usefulness of two psychometric scales in Swedish patients with severe dental fear. *Community Dent. Oral Epidemiol.,* **13**, 70–74.

Bernstein, D. and Kleinknecht, R. (1982). Multiple approaches to the reduction of dental fear. *J. Behav. Ther. Exp. Psychiatry,* **13**, 287–292.

Corah, N. (1973). Effect of perceived control on stress reduction in pedodontic patients. *J. Dent. Res.,* **52**, 1261–1264.

Corah, N., Gale, E. and Illig, S. (1979a). Psychological stress during dental procedures. *J. Dent. Res.,* **58**, 1347–1351.

Corah, N., Gale, E. and Illig, S. (1979b). The use of relaxation and distraction to reduce psychological stress during dental procedures. *J. Am. Dent. Assoc.,* **98**, 390–394.

Eiser, C., Patterson, D. and Eiser, J. (1983). Children's knowledge of health and illness:

implications for health education. *Child Care, Health Dev.*, **9**, 285–292.

Ellis, S. (1996). Response to intravenous midazolam sedation in general dental practice. *Br. Dent. J.*, **180**, 417–420.

Fassler, D. (1980). Reducing preoperative anxiety in children. *Patient Couns. Health Educ.*, **2**, 1304.

Fenlon, W., Dobbs, A. and Curzon, M. (1993). Parental presence during treatment of the child patient: a study with British parents. *Br. Dent. J.*, **174**, 23–28.

Gale, E. and Ayer, W. (1969). Treatment of dental phobias. *J. Am. Dent. Assoc.*, **8**, 130–134.

Gaudio, D. and Nevid, J. (1991). Training dentally anxious children to cope. *J. Dent. Child.* **58**, 31–37.

Ghose, L., Giddon, D., Shiere, F., et al. (1969). Evaluation of sibling support. *J. Dent. Child.*, **36**, 35–49.

Hakeberg, M. and Berggren, U. (1992). Changes in sick leave among Swedish dental patients after treatment for dental fear. *Community Dent. Health*, **10**, 23–29.

Hall, H. and Edmondson, H. (1983). The aetiology and psychology of dental fear. *Br. Dent. J.*, **154**, 247–252.

Hawley, B., McCorkle, A., Witteman, J., et al. (1974). The first dental visit for children from low socio-economic families. *J. Dent. Child.*, **41**, 376–381.

Herbertt, R. and Innes, J. (1979). Familiarisation and preparatory information in the reduction of anxiety in child dental patients. *J. Dent. Child.*, **46**, 319–323.

Howitt, J. and Stricker, G. (1965). Child patient responses to various dental procedures. *J. Am. Dent. Assoc.*, **70**, 71–74.

Ingersoll, B., Nash, D., Blount, R. and Gamber, C. (1984a). Distraction and contingent reinforcement with pediatric dental patients. *J. Dent. Child.*, **51**, 203–207.

Ingersoll, B., Nash, D. and Gamber, C. (1984b). The use of contingent audiotaped material with pediatric dental patients. *J. Am. Dent. Assoc.*, **109**, 717–719.

Jackson, C. and Lindsay, S. (1995). Reducing anxiety in new dental patients by means of a leaflet. *Br. Dent. J.*, **179**, 163–167.

Kaufman, E., Weinstein, P. and Milgrom, P. (1984). Difficulties in achieving local anaesthesia: a review. *J. Am. Dent. Assoc.*, **108**, 205–208.

Klesges, R. and Malott, J. (1984). The effects of graded exposure and parental modeling on the dental phobias of a four-year-old girl and her mother. *J. Behav. Ther. Exp. Psychiatry*, **15**, 161–164.

Lamb, D. and Strand, K. (1980). The effect of a brief relaxation treatment for dental anxiety on measures of state and trait anxiety. *J. Clin. Psychol.*, **36**, 270–274.

Lindsay, S. J. E., Humphris, G. and Barnby, G. (1987). Expectations and preferences for routine dentistry in anxious adult patients. *Br. Dent. J.*, **163**, 120–124.

Melamed, B., Weinstein, D., Hawes, R., et al. (1975). Reduction of fear-related dental management problems with use of filmed modelling. *J. Am. Dent. Assoc.*, **90**, 822–826.

Melamed, B., Yurcheson, R., Fleece, E., et al. (1978). Effects of film modelling on the reduction of anxiety related behaviour in individuals varying in level of previous experience in the stress situation. *J. Consult. Clin. Psychol.*, **46**, 1357–1367.

Miller, M., Murphy, P. J. and Miller, T. (1978). Comparison of electromyographic feedback and progressive relaxation training in treating circumscribed anxiety stress reactions. *J. Consult. Clin. Psychol.*, **46**, 1291–1298.

Nelson, W. (1981). A cognitive–behavioural treatment of disproportionate dental anxiety and pain: a case study. *J. Clin. Child Psychol.*, **15**, 79–82.

Ning, L. and Liddell, A. (1991). The effect of concordance in the treatment of clients with dental anxiety. *Behav. Res. Ther.*, **29**, 315–322.

O'Shea, R., Corah, N. and Thines, T. (1986). Dental patients' advice on how to reduce anxiety. *Gen. Dent.*, **11**, 44–47.

Rankin, A. and Harris, M. (1984). Dental anxiety: the patients' point of view. *J. Am. Dent. Assoc.*, **109**, 43–47.

Roberts, G., Gibson, A., Porter, J., et al. (1979). Relative analgesia: an evaluation of the efficacy and safety. *Br. Dent. J.*, **146**, 177–182.

Rosengarten, M. (1961). The behaviour of the pre-school child at the initial dental visit. *J. Dent. Res.*, **40**, 673.

Schurrs, A., Makkes, P. and Duivenvoorden, H. (1995). Attendance pattern of anxiety-treated patients: a pilot study. *Community Dent. Oral Epidemiol.*, **23**, 221–223.

Shaw, A. and Niven, N. (1996). Theoretical concepts and practical applications of hypnosis in the treatment of children and adolescents with dental fear and anxiety. *Br. Dent. J.*, **180**, 11–16.

Smith, T., Getz, T., Milgrom, P., et al. (1984). Evaluation of treatment at a dental fears research clinic. *Spec. Care Dent.*, **7**, 130–134.

Stokes, T. and Kennedy, S. (1980). Reducing child uncooperative behaviour during dental treatment through modelling and reinforcement. *J. Appl. Behav. Anal.*, **13**, 41–49.

Thrash, W., Marr, J. and Boone, S. (1982). Continuous self-monitoring of discomfort in the dental chair and feedback to the dentist. *J. Behav. Assessment*, **4**, 273–284.

Venham, L. (1979). The effect of mother's presence on child's responses to dental treatment. *J. Dent. Child.*, **46**, 219–225.

Veerkamp, J., Gruythuysen, R., van Amerongen, W., et al. (1993). Dental treatment of fearful children using nitrous oxide. Part 3: anxiety during sequential visits. *J. Dent. Child.*, 175–182.

Weinstein, P. and Nathan, J. (1988). The challenge of fearful and phobic children. *Den. Clin. North Am.*, **32**, 667–692.

Wright, G., Alpern, G. and Leake, J. (1973). The modifiability of maternal anxiety as it relates to children's cooperative dental behaviour. *J. Dent. Child.*, **40**, 265–271.

Chapter 7

Pain

The possibility that a visit to the dentist will be painful is an important consideration for many patients. It is often cited as a reason for both avoidance and anxiety. It is not an unrealistic concern. Depending on how it is measured, up to 77% of patients report that they feel some pain during their visit (Klepac et al., 1980a; Acs and Drazner, 1992). However, it seems that some dentists do not appreciate the importance of this factor for patients. In one survey of 20 dentists, 16 denied that their patients experienced any pain. One dentist stated 'Only once in every five years do I have a patient who has pain' (Dangott et al., 1978). The reason for this discrepancy is not clear, but it may be because some dentists assume that modern analgesics and technical equipment are adequate to eliminate pain completely, or that many dentists believe that patients' reports of pain are not credible (Murtomaa et al., 1996).

The aim of this chapter is to explore some of the research on pain and pain relief. The first section outlines the basic ideas behind modern theories of pain. Ways of measuring pain are considered in the second section. Consideration of these ideas is important for the understanding of psychological approaches to pain relief, which are considered in the third part of the chapter.

Taken together, these studies demonstrate the fallacy of the distinction that is often made between the mind and the body, between anatomy, biochemistry and physiology on the one hand and psychology and sociology on the other. While this distinction between the biological and the behavioural sciences has certain advantages, it can lead to some misleading assumptions. It is certainly not a useful approach where pain is concerned.

The experience of pain

The problem with taking a purely biological approach to pain is that it does not provide an adequate explanation for many observations. One assumption that follows from a biological view is that the magnitude of an injury should show a close correspondence with the amount of pain experienced. While this may often be the case, there are so many exceptions to the rule that it must be seen as an oversimplification. Beecher (1946) made some critical observations during the Second World War while he was treating soldiers wounded in battle. To his surprise, he found that around 60% of the soldiers who had been severely wounded reported only slight pain or even no pain at all. In contrast, during his civilian practice, where patients had received similar injuries because of surgery, virtually all reported severe pain.

At first, Beecher considered the possibility that the soldiers were in fact *feeling* much pain but were unwilling to *report* it, perhaps because this would be inconsistent with their views of themselves as stoic and uncomplaining. However, this did not seem to be an adequate explanation, since the soldiers did complain loudly about the relatively slight pain involved in injections. Beecher concluded that it was not necessarily the magnitude of an injury that was significant but, rather, the circumstances in which it occurred. In fact, readers who have participated in sports may have had less traumatic but similar experiences: athletes sometimes find that although they sustain an injury during a game, they do not notice it until the competition has finished. Similar surprises can be found in dentistry. One would expect, for example, that larger gauges of needles used for injections would result in more pain than smaller gauges, yet when Fuller et al. (1979) tested this, no differences in the amount of pain felt with 25G, 27G or 30G needles could be found.

The puzzle of these observations is complicated further by observations about *when* pain occurs. From a biological view, no pain would be expected when there is no injury, and every injury should result in pain. However, there are reports of quite severe injuries being suffered with little pain, as in some religious ceremonies in India where large steel hooks are inserted in the back muscles. At the height of the ceremony, the participants are suspended by these hooks but they seem to tolerate these injuries with little discomfort (Kosambi, 1967). Conversely, there are occasions when people experience pain without recent injury, as in phantom limb or phantom orofacial pain. Some patients who have a tooth extracted complain of pain in the location where the tooth had been removed; pain that is persistent, long-term and difficult to relieve (Marbach, 1996).

Gate Theory

Observations such as these render purely anatomical and physiological explanations of pain unsatisfactory. Perhaps the most successful approach is Melzack and Wall's (1982) Gate Theory. They suggest that the experience of pain involves not only the physical sensations resulting from an injury but also the emotional and evaluative reactions to these sensations. Signals from an injured site run to the dorsal horn of the spinal cord which acts like a kind of gate between peripheral fibres and the brain. The gate is opened (i.e. the dorsal horn cells are excited) by small fibres from the site of the stimulation and closed by other large inhibitory fibres from the same site.

These do not provide the only influences on the gate. It is also affected by fibres from the brainstem reticular formation which serve to excite or inhibit the dorsal horn cells. Reticular formations are in turn also affected by cortical activity, so that past experiences, anxiety, attention and the meaning of the situation influence the opening and closing of the gate. Thus this model provides an explanation of why a patient who has had painful dental experiences in the past or who expects much pain could actually experience more discomfort.

Components of pain

Melzack and Wall make a distinction between three components that contribute to the experience of pain. The first component is the *sensory–discriminative* which determines the perceptual information received by an individual. Such information includes the location, magnitude and timing of the stimulus. The second is the *affective–motivational* component, which provides the motivation to act as a result of this information. The third *cognitive–evaluative* component is affected by past experiences and expectations. Taken together, these interact to determine how much pain a person feels and how he or she will react to it.

Melzack and Wall argue that the sudden loss of a limb through amputation removes not only the excitatory fibres running from the injury but also the inhibitory ones, so that the gate may remain permanently open. This could explain why people who have phantom limb pain may feel the discomfort involved in the injury that led to the amputation rather than the amputation itself. It also accounts for why limb loss through leprosy, where the process is much more gradual, does not lead to phantom limb pain. For the Second World War soldiers seen by Beecher, being injured on the battlefield had positive connotations, in that it meant that they would be rested away from the fighting and were less likely to be killed. For civilian patients, a similar operation was life-threatening and a disruption to their normal routine.

Minimal tissue damage can cause severe pain if the signals from the brain open the gate wider than usual. Patients could be very sensitive to any slight tissue damage if they were very anxious or fearful of it.

What might seem to be painless to one patient may be very painful to another. Gate Theory can be used to explain some data collected by Burstein and Burstein (1979) on dental patients' responses to injections. Before the treatment, they asked patients to indicate how much pain they had experienced from injections in the past and how much they expected on this occasion. After treatment, the patients were again interviewed, this time being asked how much pain they had actually experienced. Gate Theory would predict significant correlations between these measures, and this is what the Bursteins found: memory and actual experience correlated 0.52, expectation and experience 0.80.

Implications of Gate Theory

The important point here is that physiological, psychological and situational factors interact to produce what a person experiences. This has three important implications.

Psychogenic versus somatogenic pain

One implication involves the traditional distinction between somatogenic and psychogenic pain. Somatogenic pain refers to pain which has a describable 'objective' basis, such as a bone fracture or appendicitis. A pain is said to be psychogenic if there is no discernible tissue damage: the idea here is that the pain's aetiology can be found in the psychological and not the physical state of the patient. According to this approach, pain is either psychogenic or somatogenic. Gate Theory suggests a somewhat different approach, as represented in Figure 7.1. Here, every pain is considered to have both psychogenic and somatogenic components, although one or the other may predominate for any individual in a particular situation (Dworkin et al., 1978).

Previous learning

A second implication of Gate Theory is that the experience of pain depends, in part, on previous learning. This was demonstrated long ago by Pavlov during his work on classical conditioning. Normally, dogs react strongly when an electric shock is applied to one of their paws. Pavlov was able to show that they could be taught to react with apparent pleasure if he consistently presented food after each shock. The dogs would salivate and wag their tails each time they were shocked, showing no aversive reactions. What was once painful came to be a positive event: a signal that food was about to be given. Interestingly, when Pavlov changed the site of the shock from one

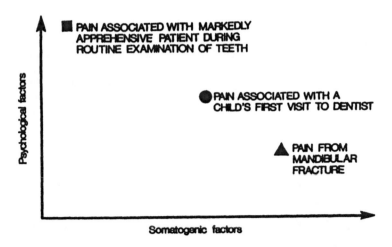

Figure 7.1. According to Gate Theory, all pain has both psychogenic and somatogenic influences, although one or the other may predominate. From Dworkin et al. (1978), with permission.

paw to another, it again elicited a violent response, indicating that the learning was locally determined.

It seems that learning about pain also occurs in humans. Many doctors have noted that reactions to painful stimuli often 'run in families'. Although it is difficult to distinguish between biological and environmental influences, parents and their children seem to react in similar ways. Perhaps children react like their parents because they are genetically similar or because their parents 'teach' them to react in certain ways, or both.

Research
A third implication of Gate Theory concerns research. Since the meaning of a situation has such an important influence on pain, the results of experiments on pain relief undertaken in the laboratory may not apply to the clinical situation. Laboratory-induced pain differs from clinically induced pain in several ways. It is short-lived and can be stopped on request, but clinical pain can be persistent, beyond the patient's control and often accompanied by high levels of anxiety. In the laboratory, pain is induced by stimuli which are novel (e.g. electric shocks, heat or cold water), whereas patients often have prior experience with clinical pain, either directly or through observations of others' reactions. Where attempts have been made to predict postoperative need for analgesia, patients react differently in the laboratory than they do on a hospital ward (Parbrook et al.,

1973). Another finding that suggests that the two types of pain are different is that morphine, which is very effective in reducing pain for clinical patients, is often ineffective in reducing laboratory-induced pain. Thus, it is important that techniques for pain relief that have proved successful in the laboratory be validated in clinical settings before they can be recommended with any confidence.

Measuring pain

Before discussing psychological interventions, it is first necessary to consider how pain could be measured. The basic problem here is that pain is a private experience, one that cannot be directly seen or felt by anyone else. Thus, some kind of indirect method must be used. Physiological, self-report and behavioural methods are three possibilities.

Physiological measures

Several physiological indices of acute stress have been employed. The level of corticosteroids in the blood, heart rate, respiration rate and the amount of perspiration are some measures. The amount of perspiration is measured by the Galvanic Skin Response: the resistance between two electrodes placed a set distance apart on the skin. The Palmar Sweat Index concerns the number of open sweat glands: a piece of sticky tape is placed over a finger and then this is removed and examined under a microscope. While there is no reason to believe that these physiological measures are any less valid than those listed below, it is important to point out that there is often a low correlation between different physiological measures (Leiderman and Shapiro, 1975).

Self-report measures

The most frequently used self-report method is some version of a 10-cm line with extremes marked at either end (such as 'the pain is as bad as it could be' and 'I have no pain'). This is called the Visual Analogue Scale or VAS. Patients are asked to place an 'x' somewhere between the extremes to indicate the degree of pain they experience. Then it is a simple procedure to measure the distance from one end of the scale to give a quantitative score (Scott and Huskisson, 1976).

Those who have used this technique have worked on the assumption that, because the scale is marked privately, it provides an accurate indication of patients' feelings, being relatively unaffected by what they believe should be expressed to others. However, the validity of this assumption is not clear. For example, different cultural groups express their pain differently, with some groups reporting more than others. People with a Northern European background tend to express their pain less readily than those from Latin countries. Even if a patient fills out the scale unobserved, such differences could still be expected to be operating. Personality characteristics are also associated with how much pain a person reports, with some people being more willing than others to express discomfort.

The McGill Pain Questionnaire

The McGill Pain Questionnaire or MPQ (Melzack, 1975) was designed to measure severity of pain along the three dimensions suggested by Gate Theory. Patients are asked to choose adjectives from a total of 20 lists which best describe the pain. Some lists refer to sensory aspects, others to the affective and evaluative ones, as shown in Table 7.1. Within each list the adjectives are rank-ordered such that a choice of, say, 'pounding' would be given a higher score than 'flickering' or 'quivering'. The amount of pain a person feels can be quantified by both the number of adjectives chosen and the weighting given to each one.

Table 7.1. Some of the lists of adjectives from the Melzack Pain Questionnaire. Patients are asked to choose those words that best describe their pain.

Sensory		Affective	Evaluative
Flickering	Sickening†	Tiring	Annoying†
Quivering	Suffocating	Exhausting*	Troublesome
Pulsing			Miserable
Throbbing†			Intense*
Beating			Unbearable
Pounding*			

* Words often chosen by women to describe labour.
† Words often chosen by patients to describe toothache.
From Dworkin et al. (1978), with permission.

Some examples of how different groups of patients respond to the questionnaire are also shown in Table 7.1. Many dental patients describe toothache as 'throbbing' on a sensory list, as 'sickening' on the affective and 'annoying' on the evaluative (Dubuisson and Melzack, 1976). In contrast, childbirth is often called 'pounding', 'exhausting' and 'intense' (Melzack et al., 1981). Van Buren and Kleinknecht (1979) asked patients who had a tooth extracted to fill out the MPQ on three occasions: the evening after the extraction and on the next two days. They found that the sensory and evaluative components showed a decrease in intensity, but the affective component remained about the same.

This is a most interesting approach to pain measurement and is becoming increasingly popular. Part of its attraction is that it might be possible to tailor pain relief techniques to particular individuals. A patient who scores highly on the sensory dimension might be given a different kind of treatment from one whose pain is mainly affective. It might also be possible to use the results in making a diagnosis. Work by Grushka and Sessle (1984) suggests that the MPQ could be used to distinguish pain originating from a reversibly inflamed tooth pulp and pain from an irreversibly inflamed or necrotic pulp. Thus MPQ results could be useful to the clinician if there is uncertainty about the vitality of the tooth. However, such an approach is in its infancy and would benefit from further study.

Behavioural measures

Non-verbal signs
Another kind of approach to measurement relies upon the behaviour of the patient. Darwin suggested that facial expressions are largely genetically determined, and different people from different cultures throughout the world show similar expressions for anger, fear, pain, and so on (Ekman, 1973). Non-verbal signs such as grimacing or tightening of the muscles during a dental procedure could indicate pain.

There is some interesting work on the possibility that there is a reciprocal relationship between experienced pain and facial expressiveness. That is, people may use their expressions to indicate to others *and to themselves* how much pain they feel. There are two studies of interest here, both of which involved giving electric shocks. Kleck et al. (1976) were interested in how people would react if they knew they were being watched, as compared to when they believed they were alone. Many people from Western cultures believe that they should not exhibit too much distress when others are present, so Kleck hypothesized that people who believed themselves to be observed would show fewer indications of pain than those who believed themselves to be alone.

In fact, everyone was videotaped so that their expressions could be monitored. As predicted, those who knew they were being watched showed less distress than those who believed themselves to be alone, indicating that expressiveness is open to social influence. However, this was only half the story. The people in the experiment were also asked to rate the painfulness of the shocks, and their skin conductance was measured. Those who were told that they would be observed gave lower pain ratings and were less physiologically aroused. Skin conductance is not easily brought under control, so there was little chance of 'faking' on this measure. In other words, being observed actually seemed to result in less pain. Other research (Lanzetta et al., 1976) suggests that this process may be due to differences in proprioceptive feedback from facial muscles.

Requests for analgesia

Instead of looking for non-verbal signs of pain, patients' requests for analgesia could be monitored. This might provide an objective measure of subjective feelings. Unfortunately, there are problems here too, since requests for analgesia, like pain rating scales, seem to be influenced by cultural and personality factors. It seems that extraverts are more likely to voice their feelings about pain and request pain relief than are introverts (Bond, 1980).

Staff responses

An alternative approach would be to monitor the amount of analgesic given by staff. Nurses, for example, could be expected to be very competent in recognizing the signs of pain due to their wide experience. Bond and Pilowski (1966) took self-report measures of pain using 10-cm scales, and then monitored patients' requests for analgesia and the responses of the nursing staff. They found that the perception of pain did not always result in a request for medication, requests when made did not always lead to administration by staff, and the strength of the medication when it was given was not proportional to the level of pain. The sex of the patient seemed particularly relevant (Table 7.2). Nursing staff were much more likely to take the initiative with female patients in administering analgesics and more likely to refuse requests from male patients. The suggestion is that cultural expectations were operating: the nurses may have believed that men should be able to tolerate more pain than women.

Table 7.2. Pattern of administration of analgesic drugs to men and women in radiotherapy wards: drugs requested and given during one week.

	Men	Women
Number of patients	15	12
Number of occasions drugs given at patient's request	23	28
Number of occasions drugs given on initiative of nurses	1	22
Number of occasions on which nurses refused patient's request for drugs	18	0

From Bond (1979), with permission.

Impact on lifestyle
This type of measure is more suited to the effects of chronic than acute pain. For general dental practitioners it could form part of the assessment for patients with temporomandibular joint problems. Chronic discomfort can pervade a person's lifestyle, such that activity is restricted and attention is almost permanently focused on the pain. Marital satisfaction, social interactions, recreational activities and employment could all be affected (Pearce and Erskine, 1989). The Sickness Impact Profile (Bergner and Bobbitt, 1981) provides scores on several dimensions, including emotions, work, sleep, eating and recreation.

Alleviating pain

These difficulties with the measurement of pain illustrate the complexity of the phenomenon. They also present problems for pain control research. One important problem concerns the finding that physiological, self-report and behavioural indices of pain do not always correlate with each other. As with the measurement of anxiety, it may be important to consider all three aspects when testing the efficacy of a technique for relieving pain.

According to Gate Theory, the sensory–discriminative, affective–motivational and cognitive–evaluative components contribute to the experience of pain. Modification of any of these would be expected to reduce the distress felt by a patient. The techniques outlined below are grouped under these three headings, although it should be said that some methods, such as relaxation and hypnosis, may be operating on more than one component at the same time.

Pain and anxiety

The contribution that anxiety makes to pain is not altogether clear. It seems most useful to consider pain and anxiety as interdependent, such that one can lead to the other. There is some evidence that dentally anxious patients are more sensitive to dental pain than non-anxious patients (Klepac et al., 1980b). When Lautch (1971) attempted to find ways of distinguishing between phobic and non-phobic patients, he found that phobic patients had a pain threshold level some 28% below the non-phobics. While it is not possible to say that lower sensitivity causes anxiety, it seems that there is an association between the two.

Thus it is no coincidence that some of the techniques discussed below have already been discussed in the previous chapter on relieving anxiety. Since anxiety is one of the contributing factors to pain, and pain to anxiety, a reduction in one should lead to a reduction in the other. Thus a frightened patient may benefit from these methods both by a decrease in distress due to anxiety and by a decrease in distress due to pain.

The sensory–discriminative component

There are several techniques that affect this component of pain. The aim of surgical procedures is to destroy neural pathways that carry impulses from the injured site. Pharmacological techniques provide short-term relief. Novocaine works by blocking nerve conduction, while morphine seems to be effective because of its similarity to enkephalins, endogenous narcotic-like substances.

The placebo effect

In studies on pain relief, it is important to include a group of people who do not receive the active treatment but instead receive an equally plausible alternative. This is to control for 'placebo effects', which are those effects of a procedure that are not due to the treatment itself, but rather to the circumstances surrounding it. These include the warmth and enthusiasm of the therapist (Gryll and Katahn, 1978), the patient's hopes and expectations that he or she will get better and the mechanics of administering the treatment (e.g. an injection or the taking of pills). Placebo effects have been shown in most areas of patient care, such as surgery, psychotherapy and the alleviation of pain (Shapiro and Morris, 1978). Figure 7.2, for example, shows the percentage of cancer patients reporting at least 50% pain relief from morphine or saline solution. There was a substantial effect from saline solution alone and the time–effect curve mimicked that of morphine (Houde et al., 1960). If there were no control groups in pain relief studies, any decreases in pain could be due to such circumstances as the attention given to the patients or simply the suggestion that the treatment will be effective.

How do placebos work?

Although the results shown in Figure 7.2 are not unusual, they are often misinterpreted. Many people believe that the placebo effect occurs for most people most of the time. This is not the case. On average, about 35% of patients obtain relief, but this varies from 0 to 100% depending on the disease and situational factors such as the patients' and dentists' beliefs about the efficacy of treatment. Personality traits and demographic characteristics (such as age and sex) are not consistently related to whether an individual responds to a placebo.

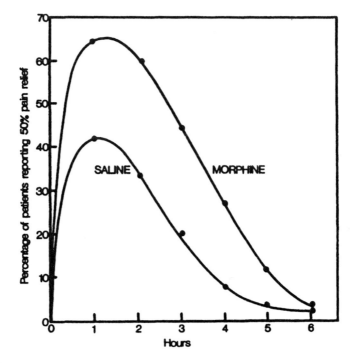

Figure 7.2. Percentage of patients reporting at least 50% pain relief over a six-hour period from 10 mg morphine sulphate or sterile saline. From Houde et al. (1960), with permission.

When placebos are effective, though, what processes are involved? One theory relies on classical conditioning. In some studies by Pavlov, dogs were given morphine and, as in the case of food and salivation, many of the animals came to show a response to morphine before they were given an injection. Perhaps the placebo effect operates in a similar way in humans: patients might feel better because this is a conditioned response to taking medication.

Another possibility has to do with selective attention. In most illnesses, the amount of discomfort varies, so a patient will feel better at some times than at others. This is certainly true of the discomfort after an extraction. Placebo effects could occur if patients became more aware of the times they did feel better and paid less attention to the times when they felt unwell.

Yet another suggestion is that patients may come to interpret their sensations as less unpleasant following a dentist's advice. Gate Theory postulates that the experience of pain is influenced by anxiety. When a dentist says that a pain reliever will reduce discomfort after an extraction – implying that discomfort is to be expected and will respond to medication – anxiety could decrease and the gate close.

On a physiological level, placebos may work through the release of endorphins (endogenous morphine-like substances) into the body. This suggestion has been tested by the administration of naloxone, an opiate antagonist which blocks the opiate receptor sites. What happens to the placebo effect when naloxone is given? Levine et al. (1978) studied patients whose impacted wisdom teeth were to be removed. Two hours after surgery, all patients were given a placebo and then, after a further hour, either placebo or naloxone. As expected, those patients who were given naloxone reported greater pain than did those given a placebo. Although this study suggests that the analgesic effect of placebos is based on endorphins, it does not answer the interesting question of how the message 'Take this, it will make you feel better' from a trusted dentist is translated into the release of endorphins.

The affective–motivation component

This component refers to the ways that people react to the sensory information they receive. A patient could react with much distress if the information was taken as a threat to his or her well-being, a threat which could not be overcome or tolerated. If the information could be considered more neutrally, without affective connotations, a patient might feel that he or she could cope with the situation in some way. The aim would be to encourage the latter kind of reaction while reducing the former. In this section, two techniques that have been shown to be useful in this way are discussed: distraction, and giving the patient some control over the dentist's behaviour.

Distraction

The idea behind the use of distraction is that patients can be provided with ways of coping with their experiences. Instead of dwelling on the sensory input, they can shift their attention away to some other kind of stimulus. One of the earlier studies in this area involved what is called audio-analgesia. Gardner and Licklinder (1959) reasoned that one of the causes of pain and anxiety in dental patients was the grinding noise of the drill. The noise was thought to raise apprehension and increase tension. They arranged for their patients to have some means of masking this noise, being given a choice of white noise (a hissing sound containing a wide range of frequencies) or music. The patients could also control the volume level. In a series of 387 patients, all of whom received cavity preparations and all of whom had previously required gas or local anaesthetic, completely effective analgesia was found for 63%. Adequate analgesia was produced in 25%, while for only 12% was the technique not successful. This method was also effective in reducing pain during extractions.

Other reports of audio-analgesia have supported this technique, though rarely with such significant results. There is some evidence that it is important that patients be *told* that attending to the white noise or music will be effective in reducing their pain. Without this suggestion the method may not be successful (Anderson et al., 1991). Whereas Gardner and Licklinder suggested that audio-analgesia works by masking the noise of the drill, it seems more likely that it is effective because it distracts the patients' attention away from the dentist's drilling.

Another method for distracting patients is to ask them to perform some kind of mental task during treatment. It may be particularly useful to encourage the imagination of pleasant and refreshing scenes rather than the performance of repetitious and dull tasks. Horan et al. (1976), for example, asked patients to listen to a tape-recording describing such relaxing scenes as walking through a lush meadow or swimming in a clear blue lake. In order to control for any placebo effects of listening to the tape and to test the efficacy of this kind of distraction over others, the patients were also asked to listen to another tape. This tape listed a series of two-digit numbers every 15 seconds and the patients' task was to imagine these numerals on a plain piece of white cardboard. On a self-report measure of distress, encouragement to imagine the pleasant scenes was the more effective technique, perhaps because it was more likely to capture the patients' attention.

It seems that many patients have learned to use such distraction techniques without a dentist's intervention. They might concentrate on another part of the body or on some object in the surgery. Thus, it might be useful to provide objects in the surgery that all patients could use to distract themselves, even if they are not showing any overt signs of pain. Hanging an interesting painting where they can see it while the dentist is working, for example, or giving them a choice of music to listen to could provide useful distractions.

Besides distraction, there are other cognitive techniques that can be used to change the emotional qualities of pain. There are indications that if patients can be encouraged to reinterpret the sensations they feel, then pain may be reduced. For example, Langer et al. (1975) asked the surgical patients in their study to try and interpret the pain they felt as optimistically as possible. They were asked to consider it as an indication that they were getting better and that it signalled an eventual improvement in their health. These and other instructions had positive effects on their recovery from the operations. As rated by nurses, for example, these patients showed less anxiety and a greater ability to cope with the postoperative period.

Enhancing control

One reason why distraction and the other cognitive strategies might be helpful is that they provide patients with some degree of control over their feelings. The idea that giving patients control over their dentists' behaviour through a stop signal has been given consistent support (Thompson, 1981). It should be pointed out that control in the sense meant here does not mean the possibility of avoiding the situation but rather the ability to influence the manner of experiencing it.

Wardle (1982) describes how she used a stop signal to reduce pain. All patients were attending a dentist for routine care, mostly fillings. Some patients were shown a stop signal – the raising of an arm – and were told that they could use it as often as they needed, whenever they wanted a rest. The dentist said that he wished them to use it at least once. For another group of patients, the dentist went about his work as usual. When the patients were interviewed after the appointment, 50% of the patients given routine care reported some pain, but only 15% of those who were told about the stop signal. In another study (Thrash et al., 1982a), significant reductions in pain and discomfort due to the injection were found. Patients were given buttons to push which lit green (signalling relative comfort), yellow (some discomfort) and red (considerable discomfort) lights. They were told that the dentist would stop when the red light was on. Whatever the stop signal, it seems particularly important that the dentist respond quickly and unambiguously to a patient's discomfort (Thrash et al., 1982b).

In these studies, few patients actually used their stop signals. It seems that the *perception* of control is the important factor, rather than the actual exercise of control. Croog et al. (1994) used this idea when preparing their patients, all of whom were due to have periodontal surgery, for postoperative pain. Those patients whose sense of control over the pain was enhanced reported fewer days of pain than those patients who were not given the intervention.

The cognitive–evaluative component

This component is primarily concerned with an evaluation of the severity of the sensory input. Is the experience only annoying or is it intense or even unbearable? Gate Theory indicates that patients' expectations about the intensity of the stimulus they will experience are very important in this respect. It has been argued that part of the difficulty that patients face in undergoing dental procedures is the way that professional dental care has come to be labelled as 'painful', so that any intense stimulation experienced in the dentist's chair is taken to be pain. Some research on this contention is discussed below, along with two further methods which seek to alter expectations about pain in dentistry, hypnosis and preparing the patient for treatment.

The word 'pain'

Several dentists have suggested that this word should be avoided whenever possible, lest the patient come to label (and feel) dental procedures as painful. In general, it is better to avoid emotive words when describing the effects of a dental procedure to a patient; for example to use the word 'restore' rather than 'drill' (Jan, 1964). It may often be possible to provide labels that do not have emotional connotations. Neiberger (1978) reports some positive results with children who were visiting the dentist to have their teeth cleaned. They were all greeted by the words 'Hello. How are you? Today we are going to clean your teeth with a magic toothbrush and toothpaste'. The number of children who cooperated with the dentist and who laughed during the cleaning was noted. Halfway through the cleaning, the dentist then added 'When I brush your teeth it will tickle and make you laugh', a comment which seemed to have an important effect on the children's behaviour.

Before this second statement, 40% of the children showed some resistance, but only 4% afterwards. Seventy-four per cent started to laugh during the second half of the appointment, compared with only 7% beforehand. Using the word 'tickle' as a label for the sensations seemed to make the cleaning enjoyable rather than distressing. One problem with this study is that the children may have become more cooperative simply because they found the cleaning to be less distressing than they expected or because they became more used to it as the appointment progressed. It would have been better to have conducted the experiment on two groups of children, one group who was told that the cleaning would tickle and one group who was not told this.

Hypnosis

Like many other complex skills, hypnosis requires some considerable training, and both patients and therapists become more proficient with practice. Although there are few well-controlled studies on hypnosis in dentistry (Kent, 1986), many case studies have indicated that much of the discomfort and anxiety associated with dental care can be alleviated by using hypnosis. The general aim of hypnosis is to help patients achieve a sense of calm well-being and a belief that they can cope with the stress of their situation (Smith, 1987).

There are a number of induction techniques, but their success seems to depend on the patient's motivation and trust in the hypnotherapist. Generally, the patient is asked to focus attention on one object, concentrating on it completely without allowing other thoughts to intrude. Coe, for example, describes how he uses a pendulum, held by the patient, in order to induce concentration and openness to suggestion:

> I want you to hold this little bob just the way I do. (Demonstrate the proper way to hold the thread.) That's it, just hold it so you can sit there comfortably and relax. Now I want you to take the attitude just for a moment or so, that that little bob is the only thing of importance to you. That's it, just focus your gaze on it, and begin trying to discover all you can about it. (It is helpful if the bob has designs, colors, or other irregularities on it.) That's it, look at it carefully, trace all around its outline, notice any geometric shapes that may be on it, like circles — squares — perhaps you can even find rectangles if you look carefully. Just try to learn everything you can about that little bob, think of it as a new and different experience, something unique, something you would like to know everything about. Notice its colors — notice how this varies from spot to spot, and how it changes — as you become more interested in the bob, you notice that in fact it becomes more the center of your attention. Your vision narrows, things in the side of your vision tend to gray out, to become less important. The bob in fact becomes the center of your attention — now watch it very closely, because in a moment it is going to begin doing something — it will begin moving back and forth, back and forth, back and forth. (1980, p. 449.)

Suggestions that are easy to follow are given first (e.g. that their attention on the pendulum has caused their eyes to become tired and the eyelids heavy). Relaxation plays an important part, with suggestions that arms and legs are becoming heavier and more relaxed. Often, patients are asked to count backwards from 10 or from 20, becoming more relaxed with each number.

When hypnotized, the patient is more open to the therapist's suggestions than in the 'waking state'. Suggestions aimed at lessening such problems as pain or anxiety are more likely to be accepted. The hypnotized person is able to listen and speak to the therapist and remains aware of who he is and what is going on around him. The patient will also reject any suggestions which he finds distasteful or unacceptable, so there is no question that the hypnotist 'controls' the patient against his will. Suggestions can be made in the hypnotic state that the patient can respond to later, when he has 'awoken', a phenomenon known as 'post-hypnotic suggestion'. In addition, a person can be shown how to hypnotize himself. Therapists regard this self-hypnosis, also known as 'autohypnosis', as very useful because the person can attain a relaxed state quickly in the absence of the hypnotist.

A trance state?

Although hypnosis was popular in the nineteenth century, it was until very recently considered with much scepticism. Part of the reason for this lack of acceptance was the problem of knowing what a hypnotic state might be. Many hypnotists characterize it as a 'trance state' — a unique form of consciousness where some critical faculties are suspended — but it is difficult to distinguish hypnotized people from those who have been coached to behave in certain ways. Many of the feats ascribed to hypnosis can be attained by most people when in the waking state. For example, stage hypnotists often suggest that a person will become rigid, so much so that he will be able to support himself with his neck on the edge of one chair and his heels on the edge of another. This looks impressive but, in fact, it can be accomplished by most fit people.

Anxiety

As mentioned earlier, hypnosis can also be used to relieve anxiety, a state which can reduce the effectiveness of analgesics. This is illustrated by the following case study (Fier, 1980):

> A twelve-year-old girl, named Mary, came to see me for routine dental care. Her general health was fine, but she reported having had a 'bad' experience in a dental office when she was 6 or 7 years old. She wouldn't tell me very much about it, and since her parents weren't present during treatment, no further information could be obtained. On further questioning Mary would only say that this dentist hurt her and nothing more. When she spoke of this experience she began shaking and was visibly upset. On her first visit Mary requested 'gas', since she had experienced it before. We began analgesia and routine excavation, but we had to stop and temporize the teeth. We couldn't find a comfortable level of analgesia for her. As soon as she relaxed, she'd pass into an

excitement stage. The stage of analgesia for Mary was almost non-existent. During her next visit, I began her hypnotic induction through visual fixation, deep breathing, and counting exercises. Using the technique of taking the patient in and out of a trance quickly and repeatedly, along with other suggestions, I was able to deepen her level of relaxation. At this point Mary's shaking stopped. Using 'eraser technique' (as a schoolteacher erases a blackboard) I facilitated Mary 'erasing' from her memory the past experience that had caused her so much discomfort. With some other suggestions, we were able to help Mary mentally transport herself to her last birthday party, which had been a very pleasant experience for her. The treatment planned for the visit was then accomplished by using local anaesthesia. At each subsequent visit, a previously spoken signal made her induction almost instantaneous. (1980, pp. 12–13)

Preparing the patient
Most patients, whether they be medical or dental, often have little idea of what is going to happen to them when they seek professional care. There is now an extensive literature that has explored the effects of preparing patients for such procedures as termination of pregnancy, gastrointestinal endoscopy, barium enemas, IUD insertion, cast removal and a variety of surgical procedures.

Sometimes the preparation can be given during a procedure. Wardle's (1982) study was mentioned earlier and involved assessing the usefulness of a stop signal for relieving pain. In another condition of the same experiment, Wardle asked the dentists to give a running commentary on their work as they performed it: what they were doing, when some discomfort could be expected and when their work would be definitely pain-free. When the amount of pain felt by this group of patients was compared with those given routine care, 50% of the latter group reported some pain, but only 22% of those who were informed as to what to expect.

More often, surgeons take steps to prepare patients well beforehand. Janis (1971) argued that patients who are informed about their operations are able to engage in what he called 'the work of worrying', a kind of inner preparation for the stress to come. Patients could plan their coping methods and rehearse them mentally if they knew what to expect. This explanation fits well with a study mentioned in Chapter 6, where the recovery of children who were given one week's notice of an extraction was quicker than the recovery of children who were told only on the day of the extraction (Baldwin and Barnes, 1966). Those given prior notice expressed a wish 'to think about it' and 'get ready for it'. Another explanation involves the reduction of anxiety. A patient who is not informed about how he or she will be treated and feel afterwards has to contend with much uncertainty, and this may increase the amount of pain experienced. A third explanation involves control: a patient who can predict what is going to happen has more opportunity to exert control than someone who has little idea about the treatment. Whatever the most suitable explanation – and perhaps all these possibilities have some truth about them – many studies have demonstrated that preparation can be effective.

Acute versus chronic pain

The distinction between acute and chronic pain is somewhat arbitrary: pain of recent onset is generally termed acute, but if it persists for more than six months it is termed chronic. Acute pain is associated with heightened autonomic arousal (e.g. increases in heart rate, blood pressure and striated muscle tone), but patients with chronic pain show habituation of autonomic signs.

From a practical point of view, acute and chronic pain have different psychological consequences. Anxiety is a common response to acute pain and the autonomic signs are consistent with the 'fight-or-flight' response. Chronic pain has more lasting effects. Depression is frequent and there can be severe curtailment of lifestyle as patients guard against exacerbating discomfort. This can result in a vicious circle: as someone becomes more careful about movements, their attention becomes increasingly focused on their bodily sensations. This in turn makes movement increasingly painful. These problems are reflected by what patients say to themselves. Phillips (1989) found that chronic pain patients would often dwell upon their discomfort (e.g. 'I wonder if they will ever find a cure for my pain?') and its effects (e.g. 'How am I going to concentrate with this awful pain?'). In such instances, pain can come to dominate a person, resulting in severe incapacity.

Chronic pain can develop after a period of acute pain, when the expected improvement does not occur despite full healing of tissue damage. Several psychological reasons have been put forward for this. Health professionals working in pain clinics would explore the possibility that a patient's maladaptive beliefs (e.g. 'I can think of nothing other than my pain') serve to exacerbate and maintain the pain because the patient constantly focuses on how he or she is feeling, rather than engaging in activity. Sometimes relatives become over-solicitous, so that they inadvertently reinforce complaints of pain.

Within dentistry, a particularly difficult condition to treat is burning mouth syndrome or BMS. Affecting perhaps 1–2% of people at any one time, it is characterized by oral burning, dry mouth, thirst, persistent altered taste perception and changes in eating habits. The difficulty does not respond well to medication (Ship et al., 1995), but Humphris et al. (1996) describe how they helped two people with BMS through psychological means. First, they took a detailed history of the patients' backgrounds. In both cases, severe life events (bereavements, financial difficulties, divorce) occurred around the time when the symptoms first appeared. Both had received extensive medical investigations but no abnormalities could be found. Humphris et al. took a series of psychological assessments and asked the patients to keep a diary of their pain levels. The main interventions consisted of challenging the patients' beliefs that their pain was a sign of serious disease (e.g. the belief that 'This continuous pain means I must have cancer') and encouraging ways of reducing stress. In both cases the amount of pain reports decreased quickly, a change which was maintained at follow-ups.

Summary

The amount of pain that a person feels cannot be predicted from knowledge of the stimulus alone. Many other factors influence the experience of pain, including the meaning of the situation, personality variables and culture. This learning could take place through the observation of friends and relatives. Gate Theory has three implications: (1) that all pains have both psychogenic and somatogenic features; (2) that the experience of pain is partly dependent on previous learning; and (3) that research on pain conducted in the laboratory may not apply to real-life situations.

These multiple influences on pain make measurement difficult. Physiological measures, such as the amount of perspiration and heart rate, provide one means of measurement. Self-reports can also be used. These include asking a patient to indicate the amount of pain he or she feels on a 10-cm line, and the McGill Pain Questionnaire, where a patient is asked to choose adjectives which best describe his or her pain. Another approach is behavioural. Here, the amount of analgesia given by staff or requested by patients could be monitored.

According to Gate Theory, psychological techniques should be effective in relieving pain for dental patients. Distraction and giving the patient some control over the dentist's behaviour are effective in alleviating pain on the affective–emotional dimension. The cognitive–evaluative component is affected by expectations about pain, so that the use of the word 'pain' itself may not always be helpful.

Hypnosis and providing patients with information about their treatment can also be effective. Whenever testing the effectiveness of a technique for alleviating pain, it is important to include a placebo control group.

Practice implications

- Pain, like anxiety, is a personal experience. Although there are verbal and non-verbal correlates of discomfort, a dentist may not always have an accurate view of the degree of pain a patient is feeling.
- There are a number of straightforward psychological techniques that dentists can use to decrease discomfort. Patients can be involved in making a choice between these methods.

References

Acs, G. and Drazner, E. (1992). The incidence of postoperative pain and analgesic use in children. *J. Dent. Child.*, **59**, 48–52.

Anderson, R., Baron, R. and Logan, H. (1991). Distraction, control and dental stress. *J. Appl. Soc. Psychol.*, **21**, 156–171.

Baldwin, D. and Barnes, M. (1966). The psychological value of a presurgical waiting period in the preparation of children for dental extraction. *Trans. Eur. Orthodont. Soc.*, 297–308.

Beecher, H. (1946). Pain in men wounded in battle. *Ann. Surg.*, **128**, 96–105.

Bergner, M. and Bobbitt, R. (1981). The Sickness Impact Profile: development and final revision of a health status measure. *Med. Care*, **19**, 787–805.

Bond, M. (1979). *Pain.* Edinburgh: Churchill Livingstone.

Bond, M. (1980). Personality and pain. In *Persistent Pain* (S. Lipton, ed.) London: Academic Press.

Bond, M. and Pilowski, I. (1966). Subjective assessment of pain and its relationship to the administration of analgesics in patients with advanced cancer. *J. Psychosom. Res.*, **10**, 203–208.

Burstein, A. and Burstein, M. (1979). Injection pain: memory, expectation and experienced pain. *N. Y. J. Dent.*, **49**, 183–185.

Coe, W. (1980). Expectations, hypnosis and suggestion in behaviour change. In *Helping People Change* (F. Kanier and A. Goldstein, eds) Oxford: Pergamon.

Croog, S., Baume, R. and Nalbandian, J. (1994). Pain response after psychological preparation for repeated periodontal surgery. *J. Am. Dent. Assoc.*, **125**, 1353–1360.

Dangott, L., Thornton, B. C. and Page, P. (1978). Communication and pain. *J. Commun.*, **28**, 30–35.

Dubuisson, D. and Melzack, R. (1976). Classification of clinical pain description by multiple group discrimination analysis. *Exp. Neurol.*, **51**, 480–487.

Dworkin, S., Ference, T. and Giddon, D. (1978). *Behavioral Science and Dental Practice.* St Louis: Mosby.

Ekman, P. (1973). *Darwin and Facial Expressions.* London: Academic Press.

Fier, M. (1980). Hypnosis in dentistry: a case history. *Dent. Surv.*, **56**, 12–13.

Fuller, H., Menke, R. and Meyers, W. (1979). Perception of pain to three different intraoral penetrations of needles. *J. Am. Dent. Assoc.*, **99**, 822–824.

Gardner, W. and Licklinder, J. (1959). Auditory analgesia in dental operations. *J. Am. Dent. Assoc.*, **59**, 1144–1149.

Grushka, M. and Sessle, B. (1984). Applicability of the McGill Pain Questionnaire to the differentiation of 'toothache' pain. *Pain*, **19**, 49–57.

Gryll, S. and Katahn, H. (1978). Situational factors contributing to the placebo effect. *Psychopharmacology*, **57**, 253–261.

Horan, J., Layng, F. and Pursell, C. (1976). Preliminary study of 'in vivo' emotive imagery on dental discomfort. *Percept. Motor Skills*, **42**, 105–106.

Houde, R., Wallerstein, S. and Rogers, M. (1960). Clinical pharmacology of analgesics. *Clin. Pharmacol. Ther.*, **1**, 163–171.

Humphris, G., Longman, L. and Field, E. (1996). Cognitive–behavioural therapy for idiopathic burning mouth syndrome: a report of two cases. *Br. Dent. J.*, **181**, 204–208.

Jan, H. (1964). General semantic orientation in dentist–patient relations. *J. Am. Dent. Assoc.*, **68**, 424–429.

Janis, I. L. (1971). *Stress and Frustration*. New York: Harcourt Brace Jovanovich.

Kent, G. (1986). Hypnosis in dentistry. *Br. J. Exp. Clin. Hypnosis*, **3**, 103–112.

Kleck, R., Vaughan, R., Cartwright-Smith, J., et al. (1976). Effects of being observed on expressive, subjective and physiological responses to painful stimuli. *J. Pers. Soc. Psychol.*, **34**, 1211–1218.

Klepac, R., McDonald, M., Hauge, G., et al. (1980a). Reactions to pain among subjects high and low in dental fear. *J. Behav. Med.*, **3**, 373–384.

Klepac, R., Dowling, J., Hauge, G., et al. (1980b). Reports of pain after dental treatment, electrical tooth pulp stimulation and cutaneous shock. *J. Am. Dent. Assoc.*, **100**, 692–695.

Kosambi, D. (1967). Living prehistory in India. *Sci. Am.*, **216**, 105–114.

Langer, E., Janis, I. and Wolper, J. (1975). Reduction of psychological stress in surgical patients. *J. Exp. Soc. Psychol.*, **11**, 155–165.

Lanzetta, J., Cartwright-Smith, J. and Kleck, R. (1976). Effects of non-verbal dissimulation on emotional experience and autonomic arousal. *J. Pers. Soc. Psychol.*, **33**, 354–370.

Lautch, H. (1971). Dental phobia. *Br. J. Psychiatry*, **119**, 151–158.

Leidertman, P. H. and Shapiro, D. (1975). *Psychobiological Approaches to Social Behaviour*. London: Tavistock.

Levine, J. D., Gordon, J. and Fields, H. (1978). The mechanism of placebo analgesia. *Lancet*, **2**, 654–657.

Marbach, J. (1996). Orofacial phantom pain: theory and phenomenology. *J Am. Dent. Assoc.*, **127**, 221–229.

Melzack, R. (1975). The McGill Pain Questionnaire: major properties and scoring methods. *Pain*, **1**, 279–299.

Melzack, R., Taenzer, P., Feldman, P., et al. (1981). Labour is still painful after childbirth training. *Can. Med. Assoc. J.*, **125**, 357–363.

Melzack, R. and Wall, P. (1982). *The Challenge of Pain*. Harmondsworth: Penguin.

Murtomaa, H., Milgrom, P., Weinstein, P., et al. (1996). Dentists' perceptions and management of pain experienced by children during treatment: a survey of groups of dentists in the USA and Finland. *Int. J. Paed. Dent.*, **6**, 25–30.

Neiberger, E. (1978). Child response to suggestion. *J. Dent. Child.*, **45**, 396–402.

Parbrook, G., Steel, D. and Dalrymple, D. (1973). Factors predisposing to postoperative pain and pulmonary complications. *Br. J. Anaesth.*, **45**, 21–33.

Pearce, S. and Erskine, A. (1989). Chronic pain. In *The Practice of Behavioural Medicine*

(S. Pearce and J. Wardle, eds) Oxford: British Psychological Society.

Phillips, H. (1989). Thoughts provoked by pain. *Behav. Res. Ther.*, **27**, 469–473.

Scott, P. and Huskisson, E. (1976). Graphic representation of pain. *Pain*, **2**, 175–184.

Shapiro, A. and Morris, L. (1978). The placebo effect in medical and psychological therapies. In *Handbook of Psychotherapy and Behaviour Change*, 2nd edn. (S. Garfield and A. E. Bergin, eds) Chichester: Wiley.

Ship, J., Grushka, M., Lipton, J., et al. (1995). Burning mouth syndrome: an update. *J. Am. Dent. Assoc.*, **126**, 843–853.

Smith, S. (1987). Hypnosis in general dental practice. In *The Dental Annual* (D. Derrick, ed.) Bristol: Wright.

Thompson, S. (1981). Will it hurt less if I can control it? A complex answer to a simple question. *Psychol. Bull.*, **90**, 89–101.

Thrash, W., Marr, J. and Boone, S. (1982a). Continuous self-monitoring of discomfort in the dental chair and feedback to the dentist. *J. Behav. Assess.*, **4**, 273–284.

Thrash, W., Marr, J. and Box, T. (1982b). Effects of continuous patient information in the dental environment. *J. Dent. Res.*, **61**, 1063–1065.

Van Buren, J. and Kleinknecht, R. (1979). An evaluation of the McGill Pain Questionnaire for use in dental pain. *Pain*, **6**, 23–33.

Wardle, J. (1982). *Management of Dental Pain*. Paper presented at the British Psychological Society Annual Conference, York.

Chapter 8

Special groups

The purpose of this chapter is to consider some groups of patients who have particular dental and personal needs. In a very real sense, of course, each patient is 'special', but it does seem useful to consider some patients as having certain problems in common. Many groups could be discussed. Patients with medical problems such as cardiac, respiratory, blood and central nervous system conditions present psychological as well as physiological challenges for dentists (Hall, 1979; Swallow and Swallow, 1980). In addition, patients who are HIV antibody positive will present ethical and confidentiality problems (Glick, 1990). There has been considerable attention given to attempts to understand the reasons why temporomandibular joint problems arise and are maintained (Dworkin, 1994; Gatchel et al., 1996).

For patients with certain medical problems, the timing of appointments could be very important. Patients with arthritis or those who have had a colostomy might require an afternoon appointment, while someone with a kidney dysfunction may prefer a morning appointment (Ettinger et al., 1979). Patients who are immunocompromised (such as children on chemotherapy) might need appointments when the waiting room is empty to reduce the risk of them picking up an infection. A child who is chronically ill and requires constant medication is under a greater risk of caries development if the medical practitioner does not prescribe sugar-free medication. A physical handicap may reduce the ability to keep teeth clean: an electric toothbrush provides a partial solution to such a problem, but perhaps the most important contribution a dentist can make in such instances is preventive advice, stressing the importance of reducing sugar in the diet and encouraging the use of fluoride supplements.

In discussing special groups of patients, it is useful to remember the distinction between impairment, disability and handicap. The term 'impairment' is used to refer to any psychological, physiological or anatomical loss or abnormality of structure or function. A 'disability' refers to the type of limitation imposed by the impairment, while the term 'handicap' refers to the difficulty a person has in fulfilling his or her roles within a family or society. Four groups of patients with varying types of impairment, disability and handicap are considered in this chapter: orthodontic patients; elderly people; people with a learning disability; and those with such mental health problems as anorexia, bulimia and depression.

Orthodontics

Research on the psychological aspects of orthodontic treatment has been conducted in three main areas. One area involves a consideration of the factors that influence the decision to seek treatment. In a longitudinal study conducted in Australia, parents and children's perception of need, dental appearance, family income and having private insurance were significant predictors of whether a child would receive orthodontic care (Spencer et al., 1995). Two other areas concern the lack of cooperation sometimes shown by children and adolescents and the psychological and social effects of treatment.

Cooperation with treatment

Most orthodontists find that some of their patients do not cooperate with treatment procedures, mainly with a refusal to wear headgear. Dental indices of the severity of malocclusion are not related to cooperation (McDonald, 1973), but the patient's perception of severity does show a relationship. Cooperative patients are more likely to be sensitive to their facial appearance and to be cooperative in other spheres, such as school (Clemmer and Hayes, 1979). El-Mangoury (1981) reports an interesting study on patients with class II malocclusions. Cooperation was measured by the amount of headgear wear, appliance maintenance, frequency of broken appointments and standard of oral hygiene. An especially relevant characteristic was the patient's concern and desire for close personal relationships – called affiliation motivation – which was the best predictor of cooperation. Those patients for whom relationships were very important were most likely to be cooperative. This could reflect a recognition of the role of appearance in relationships or it could reflect a more general tendency to try and get along with everyone, including the dentist.

One factor that may be very important for cooperation relates to the decision to seek treatment initially. Often a parent or a dentist initiates the decision to have orthodontic care, yet it is the child who has to bear the consequences. Perhaps children who receive treatment because their parents or dentist believe it to be important, but who do not share this belief, tend to be uncooperative. In other areas of health care, patients who seek help because of their own wishes are often more cooperative than those who are sent by other members of the family. Cooperation might be increased by discussing such issues with the patient at the beginning of treatment.

Social and psychological effects of treatment

There is much evidence that an individual's physical attractiveness has a significant effect on how he or she is perceived by others. A method that is frequently used in psychology experiments in this area is to present photographs to people and ask them questions concerning their expectations about those portrayed. Some photographs show physically attractive individuals while others depict less attractive people. Expectations about personality (e.g. would this person be warm and friendly or cold and aggressive?) are often measured. The question is whether a person's appearance affects other people's expectations of them. In one of the more consistently replicated findings in psychology, attractive people are seen more positively than unattractive ones.

Shaw (1981) hypothesized that children with normal dental appearance would be judged as better looking and more socially attractive than those with dental anomalies. He altered photographs to show (1) normal incisors, (2) prominent incisors, (3) a missing upper left lateral incisor, (4) severely crowded incisors, and (5) a unilateral cleft palate. Children shown these photographs were asked questions like 'If this boy (girl) was coming to your class, do you think you would like him (her) as a friend?', and adults were asked questions like 'Do you think this boy (girl) would attract friends easily?'. As predicted, children with normal incisors were rated as being more socially attractive, by both children and adults, than those shown in other photographs.

A related question is whether orthodontic treatment can affect perceived attractiveness. Korabik (1981) was able to show that it does by asking people to view photographs of the same patients taken before and after treatment: the post-treatment photographs were rated as being significantly more attractive than the pretreatment ones. In another study using the same photographs, patients were rated as being more intelligent and well-adjusted post-treatment. In both these experiments, the photos portrayed differences in facial structure rather than dentition since the mouths were closed and the configuration of the teeth was not apparent.

Although this type of research provides consistent support for a link between orthodontic treatment and perceived attractiveness, the social significance of the results is open to question. Most of the studies are rather artificial, relying on photographs, and usually no additional information about the individuals is provided. In real life, of course, the situation is very different. Dentition is only one source of information about someone. As we get to know a person better, any malocclusion becomes insignificant, and there are some studies (e.g. Shaw and Humphreys, 1982) which indicate that when further information about patients shown on photographs is given, the dentition becomes relatively insignificant. On the other hand, people can be very self-conscious about their teeth, so orthodontic care may increase individuals' self-confidence even if it has little effect on others' perceptions of them.

Self-confidence

Although one would expect that self-confidence and self-esteem would rise after treatment, this has not been shown consistently. Klima et al. (1979) examined satisfaction with body image and self-concept in three groups of children. One group was about to complete orthodontic treatment, a second group consisted of new patients, and the third group was a control, made up of children not requiring assistance. The prediction that the new group of patients would be the most dissatisfied with their appearance and would have the most negative self-concept was not supported: there were no differences between the children on the measures taken.

Since one of the main justifications for orthodontic treatment is that psychological benefits will accrue, the lack of support found in Klima et al.'s and other studies (e.g. Rutzen, 1973) have led to some questioning of the underlying assumption that people are handicapped by malocclusion. One study has addressed this specifically. Kenealy et al. (1989) took a wide range of measures of 1018 children aged between 11 and 12 years. The measures included dentists' ratings of malocclusion, teachers' ratings of attractiveness, the children's own self-ratings of attractiveness and the children's self-esteem. None of these measures correlated with each other particularly well. For example, the dentists' ratings of malocclusion correlated only 0.009 with children's self-ratings of attractiveness, and 0.032 with their self-esteem. Although it can be argued that malocclusion was relatively unimportant for these children because they had not yet reached adolescence, when self-consciousness typically increases, this study provided no evidence that, overall, children suffer from having malocclusion. Research that distinguishes between malocclusion (the impairment), the limitations it imposes (the disability) and its social effects (the handicap) may be more successful in showing an effect of orthodontic care.

Elderly patients

Many epidemiologists have noted that the proportion of patients who are elderly will increase substantially over the coming decades. This will be particularly true for those over the age of 75 years. However, it is important to note that chronological age is a poor predictor of an individual's capabilities. It is important to make a distinction between the changes that are directly due to the ageing process, and those which occur concurrently with ageing (e.g. a decline in oral health) but are not due to the ageing process itself (Gilbert, 1989). It is also important to realize that only a minority of elderly people suffer from such problems as hearing loss, senility or deterioration of vision. Surveys have shown that the facts do not support the stereotype.

The view one holds of elderly people can have important effects on how they are treated. Elderly people have the lowest dentist utilization rate of all adults. This seems to be due in part to a belief held by many older people themselves that they do not merit careful and attentive treatment. Symptoms may be interpreted as a natural part of the ageing process, rather than a result of some disease process, so that care is not sought. In many Western cultures, old age is seen as a negative attribute which can affect feelings of personal worth and self-esteem.

Views of elderly people may also affect the care given by professionals. If ageing is seen purely as a process of deterioration, then older people might be given a lower priority for allocation of scarce resources. Having pointed out the dangers of 'ageism', Berkey et al. (1996) discuss the importance of recognizing the possibility that a very elderly patient may have different treatment needs from a younger patient. Different priorities may need to be set. Patients who are over the age of 75 *may* require less intensive or aggressive interventions than younger patients, not because they deserve a lower quality of care but because they may have fewer resources to cope with major surgical reconstructions or even extensive traditional therapies. Berkey et al. list several factors that could influence clinical decision-making, including the patient's desires and expectations, the impact of the problem on the patient's own quality of life and the patient's ability to tolerate the stress of treatment.

Bereavement

Recently, there has been an increased interest in helping dentists to deal with issues related to bereavement, death and dying. In surveys, many practising dentists have indicated that education about bereavement and death ought to be included in the dental curriculum, but only a small minority have actually received training in this regard (Johnson and Henry, 1996). Bereavement counselling and bereavement therapy seek to help individuals work through many of the feelings that commonly occur after an important loss (Worden, 1982). Generally, the term 'bereavement' is used to refer to the reactions people feel after the death of a friend or relative, but it can also be used as a more general term to describe the reactions after a wide variety of losses, such as the reactions of a child who has to move school, the amputation of a limb or a total tooth clearance. Many new patients will have moved into the neighbourhood recently, and so may be experiencing a sense of loss for old friends and familiar routines.

Edentulousness

Edentulousness is increasingly becoming a condition found mainly in elderly people. This is due in part to changes in the dental profession's approach to care and in part to the lessening need for extractions due to caries. Some mention here should be made of patients' reactions to edentulousness. Many people find the prospect of having their teeth removed a disturbing one. Friedman et al. (1987, 1988) discuss how tooth loss can represent a type of disfigurement that has implications for body image and self-esteem. Such a negative reaction may be more likely if a patient is already coping with other stressful life events, if tooth loss is seen as a sign of irrevocable loss of youth and function, or if there are pre-existing problems with self-image. When wearing dentures, many patients become very self-conscious and reticent in social situations. They may refuse invitations to go out to dinner, avoid certain foods and become embarrassed if the topic is raised. Of central importance is the feeling that the appliance is a foreign object in the mouth. As one of Friedman et al.'s (1988) patients put it, '... the denture fits, I am not suffering any physical pain but part of me is gone. These are not mine, they are a dead part of myself' (p. 688). In another study (Haugejorden et al., 1993) a patient compared having to wear dentures with the loss of a job.

Many studies have been conducted on the difficulties that people often face in adapting to the wearing of dentures. The general finding is that clinical indicators of the quality of the appliance or levels of alveolar ridge resorption bear little relationship to patient satisfaction, but that patients' subjective estimates of function, absence of pain and acceptability of appearance are important factors in determining patient satisfaction and ability to adapt to the use of the appliance

(Kalk and de Baat, 1990; Willemsen et al., 1995). Although some studies (e.g. Moltzer et al., 1996) have indicated that patients who repeatedly express dissatisfaction and request many adjustments have some unusual personality characteristics, it is not possible to say that their dissatisfaction is due to their personalities – perhaps continual difficulties with eating, speaking and socializing will have negative effects on personality characteristics in the longer term (Hogenius et al., 1992). A major advance in recent years is the development of osseointegrated implants, which appear to restore patients' functional abilities and reduce distress because they are integrated psychologically as well as anatomically (Kiyak et al., 1990).

Patients with handicaps

There are many negative stereotypes in our society of people who behave 'differently' or look unusual. Those with a physical handicap or who are psychiatrically disabled are often stigmatized and avoided (Jones et al., 1984). This can have several effects on such individuals, including low self-esteem and a painful loneliness. Handicaps usually affect the functioning of families as well. The presence of a severe handicap in a newborn child can be devastating for parents and they may require considerable support.

Learning disabilities

The presence of a learning disability can be established through the use of IQ tests which are designed to measure an individual's capacity for learning, but in practice it is the ability to function in society that is of central importance. A person may have a low IQ score but be able to lead a reasonably independent life given adequate support. It is also important to point out that handicap is a matter of degree rather than of kind. There is a wide range of ability in people with learning disabilities, from those who have difficulty with basic skills such as feeding and toileting to those who can lead an independent life. While the behaviour of some people with learning disabilities can be erratic and seemingly unpredictable, most do not show such disturbances.

Severe deficits can mean that people with learning disabilities have some problems not shared by other groups of dental patients. Tooth brushing is a very complex cognitive and motor task which may be beyond their capabilities. A companion may be needed to guide them to a dentist, brush their teeth and monitor their diet. Preventive dental care is especially important, particularly if a patient will not be able to wear dentures because he or she suffers from epileptic fits. Many of the principles outlined in earlier chapters for encouraging oral health behaviours (Albino et al., 1979) and reducing disruptive behaviour (Dicks, 1974; Bloxham and Swallow, 1975) have been used with success. Regular inspections are vital, since the most severely handicapped individuals will not be able to communicate directly that they have a toothache.

Care in the community
Until recently, people requiring residential care were housed in large hospitals, but over the past decades there have been attempts to provide an environment that is as similar as possible to that of non-handicapped people. Instead of large hospitals, smaller community-based hostels are being built, and in some areas houses have been converted to allow residents to be as fully integrated into the community as their disabilities allow. This change in policy has been due in part to the recognition that living in large institutions can lead to a deterioration of abilities and in part to the recognition that it is unethical to limit a person's autonomy unnecessarily.

There has been a corresponding move to encourage general dental practitioners to treat patients with a learning disability in their offices. To this end, a few dental schools provide visits to local hostels and hospitals in order to acquaint students with the problems of treating this group of patients and to dispel any myths that might discourage the students from treating them in the future. At one dental school, for instance, two-thirds of the students had reservations about treating patients with learning disabilities, partly because they 'didn't know what to expect, had pre-conceived ideas about the patients being uncommunicative and disruptive, and were afraid that they could not handle the work emotionally or physically' (Block and Walken, 1980, p. 161). After having visited a local hospital and given restorations with the help of a well-trained dental auxiliary, 95% said that they would now be willing to treat these patients in their private practice. As one student put it, 'I became aware that unless the patients had some complicated medical problems, they are no more difficult to treat than normal patients'.

Davies et al. (1988) interviewed parents and dentists about their views on dental treatment for learning-disabled people. Many of the parents believed that regular attendance was important for the maintenance of function (30%), clear speech (20%) and aesthetics (43%), but these aspects were less important for dentists, who emphasized the prevention of periodontal disease. Both dentists and patients believed that lack of experience with people with learning disabilities was an important issue, but for the dentists the most important problems concerned the length of time that care of handicapped patients might involve, which could interfere with their efficiency. Davies et al. suggest that payment on a sessional basis could help to alleviate this difficulty.

Dentally handicapped patients
Brown (1980) has introduced the idea of the 'dentally handicapped' patient. For any one of several reasons – such as learning disability, excessive fear of dentistry, haemophilia or heart disease – a patient may be unable to receive routine dental care. In such instances, preventive care is crucial. In his study of 53 dentally handicapped children, parents cooperated in controlling diet and using electric toothbrushes and fluoride tablets. Over the course of the study there was a marked decrease in carious lesions and a corresponding increase in oral health for these children. Moreover, this programme was shown to have cost benefits, with the preventive care costing considerably less than the expected number of restorations. The involvement of parents in such a programme is clearly essential, particularly where diet is concerned.

Mental health problems

There are two reasons why dentists need to have some background in this area. First, psychological and psychiatric illnesses are much more common in the general population than is generally realized. Overall, it has been estimated that 1 in 9 males and 1 in 6 females will require an admission to hospital for psychiatric difficulties at some time in their lives (Ingram et al., 1981). Adolescence is a particularly difficult time for many people. One survey indicated that 34% of 13 to 15-year-olds had thought of suicide, 45% reported having had trouble coping with stress at home and at school, and 61% reported feeling depressed and hopeless (Waldman, 1996). Given this prevalence, it is very unlikely that any dentist will not have some distressed patients on his or her list.

A second reason why dentists need some background knowledge in this area is that people are often very reluctant to admit problems to others and to themselves. There is still a considerable stigma involved with most psychiatric and psychological difficulties. Society's rejection of people with mental health problems makes it less likely that they will seek professional help. Because of this, a dentist may be the only health care professional who will come into contact with an affected individual.

Clinical psychologists, who have an undergraduate degree in

psychology and then further training in helping people, tend to see patients who have phobias, anxiety or panic attacks or mild depression. Psychiatrists are medically trained so that they are able to prescribe a wide variety of medications for more severe psychiatric difficulties, such as schizophrenia and other psychoses. In recent years, the distinction between psychology and psychiatry has been reduced, and a psychologist and a psychiatrist often work together in a multidisciplinary team which might include nurses and social workers.

Many areas could be discussed in this section of the chapter, and more detail can be found in a wide range of introductory psychiatric texts or specialized review articles on such topics as schizophrenia (e.g. Friedlander et al, 1993a; Oxtoby and Field, 1994) or child abuse (Waldman, 1993). Two additional difficulties that may come to a dentist's attention are depression and eating disorders.

Clinical depression

Clinical depression can be distinguished from normal low mood. Most people feel 'depressed' some of the time, with feelings of low mood, some lethargy and loss of appetite. Such reactions may be due to a bereavement, failure in an examination or the end of a valued relationship. These are normal transient adjustment reactions to loss. However, clinical depression is an altogether more serious and worrying cluster of feelings, beliefs and behaviours. A person who is clinically depressed shows a general loss of vitality, loss of interest and withdrawal from social activities. There is persistent sadness and usually strong feelings of guilt and self-reproach. People often lose their appetite for an extended period of time. Although most people have thoughts about ending their own life at some point, the suicidal ideation in clinical depression may be enduring and well-developed. The person may have thought about possible means of suicide (a particularly important danger signal). Although it used to be thought that clinical depression occurred only in adulthood, it is now recognized that it can occur in children as well (Friedlander et al., 1993b). Treatments for depression include pharmacological interventions which alter the levels of certain chemicals in the brain, the encouragement of physical activity, and some psychological methods which encourage patients to reflect on the ways that they view the world (Beck et al., 1979).

Eating disorders

Much has been written about the aetiology of the eating disorders of anorexia nervosa and bulimia. Some theories emphasize the social factors that encourage young women (and more rarely young men) to attain a culturally ideal shape; others suggest that gaining control over weight provides a way for women and men to exercise control over their lives more generally, and others hypothesize that there are genetic or metabolic influences. It seems likely that there are some important social influences at work, since the prevalence of eating disorders varies over time and locale.

Anorexia nervosa refers to an aversion to food leading to severe loss of weight. Different doctors have used different criteria for diagnosing anorexia, but most agree that it is associated with a determined avoidance of food, an intense fear of becoming obese which does not decline as weight loss progresses, a preoccupation with calories, a distorted body image (perceiving oneself as fat even though severely underweight), and excessive exercising. When it occurs before puberty, there is a failure to gain weight at the expected time between 10 and 14 years, and after puberty, amenorrhoea of at least six months' duration. *Bulimia nervosa* is also associated with a preoccupation with food, but involves periods of gross overeating combined with the use of various devices such as self-induced vomiting, purging or alternating periods of overeating and periods of starvation to avoid putting on weight.

One difficulty in providing help for people with eating disorders is that they often deny that they are in need of assistance. In fact, a dentist may be the first to identify a need for treatment because of dental erosion due to repeated vomiting (Burke et al., 1996; Robb and Smith, 1996). A referral to a psychiatrist or psychologist would be appropriate, but may not be accepted at first. It is important to secure the patient's cooperation. The agency accepting the referral would aim to restore the patient's weight and help him or her examine the reasons why he or she needs to control his or her weight to such an extent.

Summary

It is often inappropriate to make generalizations about patients who share a particular condition since two people may have the same objective impairment but be disabled or handicapped in different ways. The way an individual reacts and attends to an impairment are important psychological factors during treatment. Although studies have indicated that the social and psychological effects of orthodontic work seem to be minimal for many people, it is likely that patients who are very self-conscious of the appearance of their teeth will benefit. Others may not. Some elderly people seem to take on the cultural view that they are less worthwhile than young people, and do not want to 'bother' the dentist despite the presence of severe symptoms. People with learning disabilities are sometimes unable to seek treatment themselves, relying on the vigilance of others. Dentists are often in a good position to identify people with mental health problems, since they may be the only health professionals approached.

Practice implications

- In orthodontic care it is important to assess the patient's view of the need for treatment and the psychological costs of wearing an appliance.
- Elderly patients may be reluctant to seek care. On the other hand it is important not to put pressure on them to undergo treatment when they have adapted to their oral state.
- There are many negative but unfounded stereotypes about people with learning or psychiatric difficulties. Most people with learning disabilities can be treated in private practice, but some will require additional teaching when it comes to learning new skills.
- The dentist may be the only health professional contacted by a person with a mental health problem, so it is important to be able to recognize such problems when they are present.

References

Albino, J. E., Schwartz, B., Goldberg, H., et al. (1979). Results of an oral hygiene programme for severely retarded children. *J. Dent. Child.*, **46**, 25–29.

Beck, A., Rush, J., Shaw, B., et al. (1979). *Cognitive Therapy of Depression*. London: Wiley.

Berkey, D., Berg, R., Ettinger, R., et al. (1996). The old-old dental patient. The challenge of clinical decision making. *J. Am. Dent. Assoc.*, **127**, 321–332.

Block, M. and Walken, J. (1980). Effects of an extra-mural programme on student attitudes towards dental care for the mentally retarded. *J. Dent. Educ.*, **44**, 158–161.

Bloxham, E. and Swallow, J. (1975). The dental treatment of institutionalized mentally handicapped people. *Br. Dent. J.*, **139**, 145–146.

Brown, J. (1980). The efficacy and economy of comprehensive dental care for handicapped children. *Int. Dent. J.*, **30**, 14–27.

Burke, F., Bell, T., Ismail, N., et al. (1996). Bulimia: implications for the practising dentist. *Br. Dent. J.*, **180**, 421–426.

Clemmer, E. and Hayes, E. (1979). Patient cooperation in wearing orthodontic headgear. *Am. J. Orthod.*, **75**, 517–524.

Davies, K., Holloway, P. and Worthington, H. (1988). Dental treatment for mentally handicapped adults in general practice. *Community Dent. Health*, **5**, 381–387.

Dicks, J. (1974). Effects of different communication techniques on the cooperation of the mentally retarded child during dental procedures. *J. Dent. Child.*, **41**, 283–288.

Dworkin, S. (1994). Perspectives on the interaction of biological, psychological and social factors in TMD. *J. Am. Dent. Assoc.*, **125**, 856–863.

El-Mangoury, N. (1981). Orthodontic cooperation. *Am. J. Orthod.*, **80**, 604–622.

Ettinger, R., Beck, J. and Glenn, R. (1979). Eliminating office architectural barriers to dental care of the elderly and handicapped. *J. Am. Dent. Assoc.*, **98**, 398–401.

Friedlander, A., Friedlander, I., Eth, S., et al. (1993a). Dental management of child and adolescent patients with schizophrenia. *J. Dent. Child*, **60**, 281–287.

Friedlander, A., Friedlander, I., Yagiela, J., et al. (1993b). Dental management of the child and adolescent with major depression. *J Dent. Child*, **60**, 125–131.

Friedman, N., Landesman, H. and Wexler, M. (1987). The influence of fear, anxiety and depression on the patient's adaptive responses to complete dentures. Part 1. *J. Pros. Dent.*, **58**, 687–689.

Friedman, N., Landesman, H. and Wexler, M. (1988). The influences of fear, anxiety and depression on the patient's adaptive responses to complete dentures. Part II. *J. Prosthet. Dent.*, **59**, 45–48.

Gatchel, R., Garofalo, J., Ellis, E., et al. (1996). Major psychological disorders in acute and chronic TMD: an initial examination. *J. Am. Dent. Assoc.*, **127**, 1365–1374.

Gilbert, G. (1989). 'Ageism' in dental care delivery. *J. Am. Dent. Assoc.*, **118**, 545–548.

Glick, M. (1990). HIV testing: more questions than answers. In *Controversies in Dentistry. Dental Clinics of North America* (A. Schlossberg, ed.) London: Saunders.

Hall, R. (1979). Dental management of the chronically ill child. *Aust. Dent. J.*, **24**, 334–341.

Haugejorden, O., Rise, J. and Klock, K. (1993). Norwegian adults' perceived need for coping skills to adjust to dental and non-dental events. *Community Dent. Oral Epidemiol.*, **21**, 57–61.

Hogenius, S., Berggren, U., Blomberg, S., et al. (1992). Demographical, odontological and psychological variables in individuals referred for osseointegrated dental implants. *Community Dent. Oral Epidemiol.*, **20**, 224–228.

Ingram, I., Timbury, G. and Mowbray, R. (1981). *Notes on Psychiatry*. Edinburgh: Churchill Livingstone.

Johnson, H. and Henry, R. (1996). Death, dying and bereavement education in dental schools. *J. Dent. Educ.*, **60**, 524–526.

Jones, E. E., Farina, A., Hastorf, A., et al. (1984). *Social Stigma*. New York: Freeman.

Kalk, W. and de Baat, C. (1990). Patients' complaints and satisfaction 5 years after complete denture treatment. *Community Dent. Oral Epidemiol.*, **18**, 27–31.

Kenealy, P., Frude, N. and Shaw, W. (1989). An evaluation of the psychological and social effects of malocclusion: some implications for dental policy making. *Soc. Sci. Med.*, **28**, 583–591.

Kiyak, A., Beach, B., Worthington, P., et al. (1990). The psychological impact of osseointegrated dental implants. *Int. J. Oral Maxillofac. Implants*, **5**, 61–69.

Klima, R., Witteman, J. and McIver, J. (1979). Body image, self-concept and the orthodontic patient. *Am. J. Orthodont.*, **75**, 507–516.

Korabik, K. (1981). Changes in physical attractiveness and interpersonal attraction. *Basic Appl. Social Psychol.*, **2**, 59–65.

McDonald, F. (1973). The effect of age on patient cooperation in orthodontic treatment. *Dent. Abstr.*, **18**, 52.

Moltzer, G., Van der Muelen, M. and Verheij, H. (1996). Psychological characteristics of dissatisfied denture patients. *Community Dent. Oral Epidemiol.*, **24**, 52–55.

Oxtoby, A. and Field, E. (1994). Delusional symptoms in dental patients: a report of four cases. *Br. Dent. J.*, **176**, 140–143.

Robb, N. and Smith, B. (1996). Anorexia and bulimia nervosa (the eating disorders): conditions of interest to the dental practitioner. *J. Dent.*, **24**, 7–16.

Rutzen, S. (1973). The social importance of orthodontic rehabilitation: Report of a five year follow-up study. *J. Health Soc. Behav.*, **14**, 233–240.

Shaw, W. (1981). The influence of children's dentofacial appearance on their social attractiveness as judged by peers and lay adults. *Am. J. Orthodont.*, **79**, 399–415.

Shaw, W. and Humphreys, S. (1982). Influence of children's dentofacial appearance in teacher expectations. *Community. Dent. Oral. Epidemiol.*, **10**, 313–319.

Spencer, A., Allister, J. and Brennan, D. (1995). Predictors of fixed orthodontic treatment in 15-year-old adolescents in South Australia. *Community. Dent. Oral Epidemiol.*, **23**, 350–355.

Swallow, J. and Swallow, B. (1980). Dentistry for physically handicapped children in the International Year of the Child. *Int. Dent. J.*, **30**, 1–5.

Waldman, H. (1993). Your next pediatric dental patient may have been physically or sexually abused. *J. Dent. Child.*, **60**, 325–329.

Waldman, H. (1996). Are you treating youngsters who are should be receiving mental health services? *J. Dent. Child.*, **63**, 434–437.

Willemsen, W., de Baat, C., Truin, G-J., et al. (1995). Changes in dental attitude and behaviour among Dutch adults wearing complete dentures. *Community Dent. Oral Epidemiol.*, **23**, 104–109.

Worden, J. (1982). *Grief Counselling and Grief Therapy*. London: Tavistock.

Chapter 9

Communication and consent in dental practice

In this final chapter, we turn our attention to aspects of communication in the dental setting. The first section concerns research on the verbal and non-verbal relationships between dentists and patients. The second part is a discussion of some ethical issues that arise in dentistry.

Communication

Many studies described earlier in the book illustrate that dental care is a two-way process. The three types of relationship described by Szasz and Hollender (1956) are relevant here. As outlined in Chapter 2, the mutual participation type of relationship, where the dentist and the patient share the responsibility for the patient's oral health, is usually the most appropriate model in dentistry.

Involving patients in treatment decisions

In the past, dentists often held the view that they, not the patients, were in the best position to make decisions about the type of care provided. To take the fitting of dentures as an example, Lefer et al. (1962) noted that dentists could believe that patients should be persuaded to choose appliances that complement their personality and appearance, and that any resistance shown by patients should be overcome for their own good. According to this view, the dentist is in the best position to make this aesthetic decision. Lefer et al. argued that this approach was seriously misplaced since it relies on the professional's view of what is right for a patient: a view which might not be shared by the patient him- or herself.

Lefer et al. performed a simple experiment to test the hypothesis that patients would be more satisfied with their dentures if they were involved in the choice of set-up. One group of dentists was asked to treat their patients in the traditional fashion, which was usually deciding themselves on the dentures' appearance. The other dentists were instructed to involve the patients in the choice: the patients were asked to select the size, colour and set-up of the appliance from 12 possibilities. The dentists told the patients to 'Take your time until you come to your own decision' and 'Your opinion is more important than mine'.

It soon became clear that the dentists' choices did not correspond particularly well with the patients'. For example, over 50% of the patients preferred a 'textbook' set-up, but this was given by the dentists to only 15% of the patients. In contrast, the type of denture given by the dentists 50% of the time was chosen by only 30% of the patients. In general, patients seemed to prefer set-ups that looked similar to their natural teeth. Patients who had the decision made for them made comments like 'I wish they were a little darker and longer – the way my own teeth used to look', while patients who were given the right to choose expressed their satisfaction (e.g. 'That's how I wanted to look and I've been happy with the results'). On average, those given a choice required only half as many adjustments (mean = 1.5) than those given no choice (mean = 2.9). They were less likely to complain or reject the appliance and made fewer visits for corrections.

The dentist's personality

The study by Lefer et al. indicated that involving patients in the choice of their own dentures resulted in fewer complaints. The personality of the dentist can also affect satisfaction. In another study (Hirsch et al., 1973), dental students were given a personality questionnaire designed to measure 'authoritarianism', which is a personality trait referring to the extent to which a person is power-oriented in relationships. Someone who scores high on authoritarianism tends to be obedient to those considered 'superior', but dominant over those seen as 'inferior'. The students were then asked to construct an appliance which their patients had previously been involved in selecting. At the end of the treatment, a faculty member examined the dentures to be sure that they were clinically satisfactory and that the patients' wishes had been followed. The interest was in the relationship between the students' scores on the authoritarianism questionnaire and patient ratings of the dentures.

As shown in Figure 9.1, the patients were asked to give a rating of their choice both before and after it was constructed: before treatment the patients gave ratings between 'good' and 'very good', but after treatment there was a significant difference between those assigned to high- and low-authoritarian students. The patients in the former group now reported less satisfaction than those in the latter group. It seemed that the students' personalities affected satisfaction in some way.

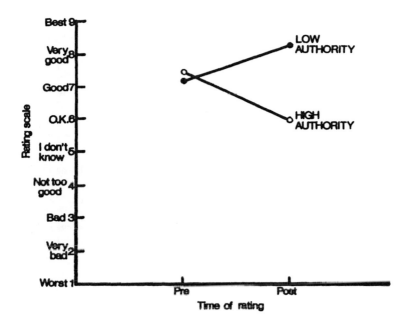

Figure 9.1. Patients' ratings of denture set-ups before and after they were constructed by high- and low-authoritarian students. From Hirsch et al. (1973), with permission.

Patients' complaints

Unfortunately, there was no follow-up of the patients in the study by Hirsch et al., so it is not possible to gauge the long-term consequences of authoritarianism. It would also have been useful to have made a recording of the consultations between students and patients so that the different ways in which the high- and low-authoritarian students related to their patients could have been specified. However, an analysis of letters of complaint sent to a dental society supports the idea that the willingness of a dentist to listen, negotiate and share responsibility with a patient is important. For example:

> The reason I went to ... is because I thought I would get my teeth done the way I wanted them done. He had long white teeth in the impression set so I told him I'd like smaller teeth and my face filled out a bit more. He became angry and said it would be better to have the pink part thin, and he didn't want to use small teeth and said they wouldn't be right for my age. I said I'd still prefer to

have smaller teeth and my face filled out more, but he became annoyed and walked out of the room. The nurse came in and dismissed me.

and:

The reason I asked ... to replace the cap on my front tooth was to improve my appearance, and I made that quite clear from the start. I told him I wanted the tooth a certain shape. Also, I wanted the tooth smooth, the same shade all over, as the old cap had a yellow splotch. When he first put in the new cap, I told him it was too narrow at the neck and not straight as it slanted towards the centre. He replied that it was natural to slant that way and his did. Then I showed him that the bottom half of the cap was blue. He said this was done because it looked more natural this way. He knew I wasn't happy about the cap but how can I get anywhere with him as he is always right and I am always wrong? (Hirsch et al., 1973, pp. 747–748).

Verbal communication

One of the more important studies in this area was conducted by Wurster et al. (1979). They examined the communication patterns between senior dental students and their child patients. The appointments were recorded on videotape and the students' and patients' behaviour was later noted: every six seconds a judge rated the kind of behaviour being shown at that moment. For the children, behaviour was rated as being cooperative (responding in a relaxed and non-fearful manner), resistant (when a child seemed to be experiencing some distress but this was not interfering with treatment) or uncooperative (resistance to the point of interfering with treatment). The students' behaviour was categorized as being directive and guiding (e.g. providing a straightforward statement of instruction while encouraging the patient), permissive (allowing any disruptive behaviour to continue unabated) or coercive (attempting to overcome disruption by threatening, ridiculing or using physical restraint). Then, Wurster examined the tapes to see how the children reacted (cooperative, resistant or uncooperative) to each of the different actions (guidance, permissiveness or coercion) shown by the students. Results indicated a 0.85 probability that direction and guidance would be followed by cooperation, a 0.67 probability that permissiveness would be followed by non-cooperation and a 0.97 probability that coerciveness would be followed by non-cooperation or resistance.

However, we cannot say from this study that direction and

guidance leads to or causes cooperation because a child may have been cooperating to begin with and a student may have been responding to this: it is possible that the students were responding to the children's behaviour, rather than vice versa. A further analysis of the tapes supported this possibility. When the communication patterns were examined from the other direction, looking to see what the students did after cooperation, resistance or non-cooperation, it seemed that the children had a significant impact on the dentists' behaviour. When the children were cooperative, the students almost always responded with directive guidance (probability 0.93), but when a child behaved in an uncooperative manner, the students usually responded with permissive or coercive behaviour (probability 0.73).

In order to say that certain behaviour on the part of the dentist *leads* to certain behaviour on the part of the child patient, it would be necessary to examine those instances when a child is being disruptive, look at how the dentist reacts, and then relate this to the child's subsequent behaviour. Do different kinds of reactions result in different kinds of behaviour? Weinstein et al. (1982) used this method in their study of dentists and their child patients. All the children were 3–5 years of age, having appointments for routine treatment. At each point in time their behaviour was categorized as being either fearful (as shown by, for example, crying, movement or protest), or non-fearful. When they were showing fearful behaviour, the dentists' responses were noted and the probability that these would be followed by continuing fear was computed. At such times, the probability that continued fearful behaviour would continue was 0.82 when the dentist was coercive, 0.55 when the dentist was coaxing and 0.48 when the dentist set specific rules for behaviour. When the dentist belittled or ignored a child, the probability of fearful behaviour continuing was also high. In contrast, when the dentist questioned the children about their feelings, or asked rhetorical questions, fearful behaviour decreased (probabilities of 0.37 and 0.26). Explanation and direction (0.30 and 0.20, respectively) were useful responses. When the dentist gave praise, specific comments like 'I like the way you keep your mouth open' were more effective than general ones, like 'Good boy' (Weinstein and Nathan, 1988). The dentist's non-verbal behaviour was also important, as discussed in the next section.

Experimental methods can be used to examine the effects of dentists' behaviour on their patients, by asking dentists to react in certain ways to disruptive or uncooperative behaviour. There is some work using this approach, where it was found that those children who were reprimanded for inappropriate or disruptive behaviour showed the most anxiety, but when the dentist was more neutral and non-evaluative the greatest degree of compliant behaviour was shown (Melamed et al., 1983).

Non-verbal communication

These studies indicate that some kinds of response to disruptive behaviour are more effective than others. However, everything a dentist says is embedded within a frame of non-verbal behaviour which serves to elaborate and modify the meaning of a statement. Generally speaking, the non-verbal aspects of conversation have a greater impact on the emotional quality of relationships, whereas verbal communication is more relevant to shared cognitive tasks and problems. Indications of friendship, assertiveness and dominance, for example, seem to depend more on non-verbal than verbal behaviour.

There are a great many non-verbal signals that influence our interactions with other people. Even the architectural features of the dentist's office can convey many messages. Besides the general decor of an office, there may be architectural barriers that prevent some patients from receiving the services they need. A narrow door, a surgery that is not large enough to accommodate a wheelchair or a great many steps are non-verbal indications that physically handicapped people have not been considered. During conversation, the way we sit, move and look are some important influences, as are the context of the encounter and the nature of past interactions. For example, eye gaze can have two distinct and almost incompatible meanings, depending on the circumstances. When two people know each other well and the circumstances are friendly, long periods of looking at each other suggest intimacy, but when issues of status are at hand, eye gaze may indicate aggression. Similarly, touching may indicate caring or dominance.

Furthermore, many non-verbal signals interact with each other. Argyle and Ingram (1972) reported that people look at each other more frequently when they are separated by a large distance than when they are close together. They suggest that eye gaze and distance can substitute for each other as signs of intimacy, so that in order to keep a constant level of intimacy, people will look at each other less often and for shorter periods of time when they are close together. An everyday example of this can be found in crowded buses: everyone is standing close together and studiously looking out of the window or at the advertisements.

Vision
Being able to see a conversational partner is not necessary for

interaction (it is possible, for instance, to talk over the telephone) but it does play an important role in most conversations. When a person is speaking, he or she will tend to look at the partner infrequently and for short periods of time, presumably because of a concern with formulating what to say. Attention is focused mainly on thinking. When a person is listening, he or she will spend most of the time looking at the speaker, showing attention to what is being said. Listeners who do not look and who do not show interest and attention are often judged to be unfriendly and distracted. Whether speaking or listening, the amount of gaze a person gives appears to affect others' perceptions of friendliness and warmth. Thus, a patient who is visually ignored by the dentist may well feel that the dentist is not especially attentive or caring.

There are several studies concerned with the role of vision in doctor–patient consultations. For example, Byrne and Heath (1980) videotaped several interviews, looking especially at the relationship between doctors' behaviour and the speaking patterns of the patients. Clearly, the patients would stop speaking – sometimes in mid-sentence – whenever the doctor looked down and began writing. Only when the doctor looked up again did the patients resume. Apparently, the patients assumed that the doctors were attending to their writing and would not be listening to what they said. Similarly, dentists may be interested to see if these ideas apply to their own work. Do patients stop describing their symptoms or difficulties when you appear to be busy with some other task?

Posture and gestures

The posture assumed by conversationalists is very important. A slight forward lean has been shown to be associated with perceptions of warmth. Closed-arm positions appear to indicate coldness or rejection while moderately open-arm positions convey warmth and acceptance. Changes in posture can convey a wealth of information. They often accompany a change in topic and can be used to signal the end of a conversation. If people are seated while talking, for instance, standing up is a clear signal that the conversation is coming to an end. Movement is also used to emphasize a point or to demonstrate an idea. The representation of size with the hands commonly occurs: people often hold them far apart when describing a large object, close together when describing something small. Facial movements comprise perhaps the most expressive non-verbal signals. Many are common to all cultures, since people of very different upbringings smile, laugh and cry in similar ways.

Posture, gestures and facial movements are some non-verbal signals that are commonly used to infer patients' anxiety or pain, but as discussed in earlier chapters, the correlations between dentists' ratings of overt behaviour and patients' self-reports of anxiety and pain are by no means perfect, and are often quite low. This may be because there is, in fact, little relationship between the two or, alternatively, that not everyone is particularly skilled at discerning inner feelings from overt behaviour. There is evidence from the medical literature that some doctors are much more adept than others in their ability to appreciate the emotions of patients, a point taken up later in this chapter.

Proximity

One way of understanding the distance that people keep between each other is in terms of 'personal space': a kind of bubble of portable territory. One method of discovering the size of this space is to observe conversationalists and then measure the distance between them. When standing or talking casually, people in our culture usually keep about 60–70 cm between them. In some other cultures, the distance is smaller. A way of testing the validity of this observation is, simply, to walk closer to someone and measure the distance at which he or she begins to move backwards. The point at which this occurs is the edge of the bubble. It seems from experiments of this type that the bubble is not round: people will tolerate more proximity at their sides than at the front or back.

The boundaries of personal space vary according to several situational factors. Intimacy of topic is one variable, as is the relationship between the participants (e.g. friends or strangers). Hall (1967) categorized proximity into four zones: Intimate (0–18 in.), Personal (18 in. to 4 feet), Social (4–12 feet) and Public (more than 12 feet). The topic of conversation and the relationship between the participants using these different zones varies. For instance, two people standing or sitting between 4 and 12 feet apart are more likely to be speaking socially than personally or intimately.

Much dental care involves the intimate zone, particularly physical contact. Weinstein et al. (1982), in their study of the effects of dentists' behaviour on the fear of their child patients discussed earlier, assessed the probabilities of continuing fear following various forms of touching. Holding and restraining increased the likelihood of fearful responses (probability 0.62 and 0.85, respectively), while patting seemed to reduce it (probability 0.30).

It is also interesting to speculate on the meaning of an oral examination and treatment for patients in this regard. Like doctors and nurses, dentists seem to have a kind of special licence to enter personal space and touch patients, but there is little evidence to indicate whether this results in uncomfortable feelings or whether patients feel completely neutral about it. The assumption that it is culturally acceptable for dentists to touch their patients cannot be taken as an indication that there are no significant meanings attached. Nurses also have the right to touch their patients, but they often find them disclosing very personal information during intimate forms of touching. Medical patients sometimes complain that they feel violated in some way when doctors physically examine them without any prior attempt to establish some rapport. Because of the link between touch and intimacy, it may be important that dentists, too, spend some time with a new patient before attempting examination in order to develop an appropriate relationship.

Teaching communication skills

Perhaps the most frequent question asked about the training of dentists in communication skills is: Why are they needed? Every dentist is, after all, a highly skilled psychologist in many ways, having had much experience with many people. Many of the abilities needed should be 'picked up' during the dental course by watching how members of staff relate to their patients and later by noting how patients react to comments and advice.

While there is some validity in these arguments, there are also indications that this kind of informal training is not always adequate. In their study of students and child patients outlined earlier, Wurster et al. (1979) asked the students to rate their confidence in their ability to cope with difficult patients. The students were given a series of hypothetical situations, such as 'Four-year-old Donna attempts to leave the chair during placement of a rubber dam'. They were asked to indicate their confidence in being able to cope with such situations on a 10-point scale ranging between 'I feel my skills are disturbingly inadequate. I do not think I am able to control this behaviour more than one time out of ten' and 'I feel my skills are completely adequate. I am able to control this behaviour whenever it occurs'. The students were then divided into high- and low-confidence groups and their actual behaviour with the patients noted. The less confident students accounted for 86% of the permissive behaviours and 95% of the coercive ones. As discussed earlier, these were the kinds of reactions associated with uncooperative behaviour on the part of the children. Indeed, the patients of the less confident students accounted for 87% of the uncooperative behaviour shown by all the children in the study. Since the children were assigned to the students without knowledge of their confidence levels, it seems unlikely that this difference was due to the children's personalities.

It is useful to consider interpersonal abilities as particular kinds of skills, much like riding a bicycle, driving a car or drilling a cavity. When first learning to drive, a person may feel awkward and unsure, but soon becomes more comfortable as the skills become automatic. A student who is about to drill his or her first cavity on a patient is likely to be anxious and unsteady, but with practice the action becomes more assured and smooth. Just as these physical skills can be taught and developed, so too can social skills. Many programmes have been developed coming under the rubric of Social Skills Training (SST) (Furnham, 1983). This approach has been used in a variety of situations from helping managers to communicate with their employees to helping doctors in their consultations with patients. Some dental schools include social skills training in their curricula, and examples of these programmes are discussed next.

Training programmes

One of the most important concepts in patient care of almost any type is called 'accurate empathy'. This refers to two complementary abilities. The first involves the ability to discern the meaning of patients' verbal and non-verbal behaviour. The second component is the ability to express the understanding gained through this sensitivity. That is, it is not only important to be able to gauge emotions but also to indicate this to the patient.

Several programmes attempt to increase dentists' accurate empathy. Jackson (1975, 1978) describes his approach in some detail. He argues that many of the comments made by dental patients have both a surface meaning and a deeper, more subtle, meaning. For example, a patient could say to a dentist who is new to a practice: 'I liked ... I went to him for 30 years, you know', or a parent could say 'Can I come into the surgery with my son?'. In his training programme, Jackson encourages students to translate such comments, looking for deeper meanings. So in the first example, the possibility that the patient is saying 'I'm not sure that I trust you' might be considered, or in the second example perhaps the parent is saying 'I am worried about my son's dental care and whether you will treat him properly'. Jackson suggests that statements referring to the amount of work required, length of treatment, size of cavity and necessity for a local anaesthetic probably reflect fears of discomfort, while comments about the equipment, age of the dentist and difficulty of the procedures frequently represent patients' concerns with technical competence.

Types of response
The next step involves a consideration of how to respond to such comments. First, a distinction is made between relevant and irrelevant responses, so that:

Patient: I see you have a new drill.
Dentist: Yes, a Siemens 242×43, a real beauty.

would be considered an irrelevant response, since it is unlikely that the patient was concerned about the name of the equipment; more likely that he was expressing some degree of anxiety about it.
Relevant responses fall into four categories:

1. Evaluative responses, which tend to make patients feel that they are being evaluated negatively or told that they should not feel the way they do, for example:

Patient: I brush my teeth and floss at least once a day and I think it is ridiculous that I have two cavities this check-up.
Dentist: Now, I never gave you any assurances that you wouldn't still have some cavities; anyway, two small cavities is a pretty good check-up. You should be very satisfied.

When this exchange is translated, it might read

Patient: I am disappointed and frustrated.
Dentist: I do not approve of you being disappointed and frustrated. You should be very satisfied.

Another example:

Patient (a child): I hate dentists. I don't want to be here. I want to go home.
Dentist: Come now. Even your little brother didn't mind his check-up. Be a good boy and open your mouth.

could be translated as

Patient: I am afraid.
Dentist: Because you are afraid I think you are both childish and bad.

2. Supportive responses, which imply that it is unnecessary for the patient to feel as he does, for example:

Patient: I am really concerned about this extraction.
Dentist: No need to be, it does not seem to be a very difficult one. It should not take more than 10 minutes.

3. Probing responses ask for more information or explanation. It is

useful to use the patient's own words if possible, for example:

Patient: I hate going to the dentist.
Dentist: What do you hate about it?

4. Understanding responses, which indicate that the dentist realizes and accepts the patient's concern, for example:

Patient: Can I come into the surgery with my son?
Dentist: You're wondering how he will react.

Such training programmes make the assumption that it is better for a dentist to act in an understanding or supportive way than to be evaluative or irrelevant. In order to test this assumption, Jackson gave examples of written conversations between dentists and patients to (non-dental) students, so that, for example, all the students saw the patient's comment:

The only reason I'm here is because this tooth is killing me, otherwise you'd never find me in a dentist's chair.

One-third saw the evaluative response:

If you had come in for regular check-ups, you probably would not be having so much pain.

another third saw the supportive response:

Don't worry, we'll look after you.

and the rest the understanding one:

It really bothers you to see the dentist.

The students were shown several such conversations and asked to make judgements about the kinds of dentists who would make such responses. The understanding and supportive dentists were said to be significantly more sensitive, altruistic and warm than the evaluative ones.

Programme evaluation

It is important to evaluate training programmes in order to measure their effectiveness. Such evaluation could be conducted by comparing students' behaviour before and after a training course or by giving the course to one group of students while another group, not given the training, serves as a comparison. Jackson used the latter approach. Half the students were given a course of three two-hour sessions describing the ideas of attending and responding, as described above. Students in the control group received no training in these ideas.

Then, all were asked to role-play a dentist who was to explain the reasons for an extraction to someone who was playing the role of a patient. This patient did not want the treatment. Their consultation was videotaped and later shown to two judges who rated the students' behaviour on a number of dimensions, including empathy, respect and genuineness. These were not the specific skills taught but, rather, more global assessments of interpersonal ability and warmth. When the ratings of the two groups of students were compared, those given the training programme were seen to be significantly more able, particularly on the scales of empathy and respect.

Another kind of training programme is described by Levy et al. (1980). The students were first given a brief description of 12 patient management skills. These skills included many of the ideas discussed in earlier chapters, such as giving positive reinforcement for cooperative behaviour, providing truthful and accurate information and informing patients of stop signals. Then, each student was observed during an actual appointment with a patient. The observer noted two kinds of management skills (e.g. information-giving and positive reinforcement) which seemed lacking for each student. These deficits were then discussed and the students were to try and improve them during subsequent appointments. When the student's behaviour in one of these subsequent appointments was monitored, there was a significant improvement in the quality of the targeted skills.

Gaining feedback

One problem that dentists face is in knowing if a consultation has succeeded or not from the patient's point of view. Few patients express dissatisfaction to their dentists directly. It is more probable that they will simply go elsewhere for their next appointment. This leaves the dentist not knowing if the patient has moved away, is content but has not attended for a long time, or has found another dentist. Some methods for increasing feedback have already been mentioned, such as asking probing questions and using non-verbal signs of interest. Some training programmes have included a formal feedback process. During training, a student might be asked to videotape a consultation with a patient and then play the tape back in the presence of peers or staff. In some programmes, the patients themselves are also present at the playbacks, so that they can contribute their viewpoints. By asking both patients and students to discuss the thoughts they had during the interview, a more complete understanding of the consultation can be achieved.

This can, however, be expensive in terms of the amount of time spent with each patient. Gershen et al. (1980) have developed an interesting alternative. They first videotaped some appointments between dentists and their patients. Then, each dentist and patient and a member of the dental school teaching staff discussed the tape in depth. This conversation was, itself, audiotaped and the participants' comments edited on to the original videotape. This meant that the appointments could be shown to dental students with both the dentist's and the patient's comments being included in the background. While this method has the disadvantage of not being tailored to each student's requirements, it is a readily available teaching aid for calling attention to the patient's feelings and concerns during treatment.

Ethical issues

To a reader new to the field of ethics, it may seem that dentists have little need to be concerned with this aspect of their practice. In the popular view, ethics is mainly concerned with such major issues as abortion and euthanasia. However, ethics is as important in dentistry as it is in medicine. Every consultation between a health professional and a patient has ethical implications. The values we hold as health professionals are crucial for practice. Being a dentist involves more than scientific curiosity and practical skills. It also involves an obligation to work towards patients' physical, emotional and social well-being. In order to meet this obligation, it is important to consider carefully the choices we make, while respecting the rights of patients, their families and wider society. Common problems encountered by general dental practitioners include the need to compromise standards because of time pressures or because a patient cannot afford the ideal treatment, finding poor treatment performed by other dentists, obtaining consent from patients who are children or who have learning difficulties, and confidentiality issues (Hasegawa et al., 1988; Osborne, 1993; Kress et al, 1995; Sfikas, 1996).

Ethical principles and rules

Moral philosophy does not necessarily *tell* dentists how to make ethically demanding choices, but it can help to clarify the important issues. Ethicists often base their understanding of ethical choices on four principles and four rules.

Philosophers distinguish between four basic principles. The first principle is *autonomy*. This term comes from the Greek 'autos' (meaning self) and 'nomos' (rule, or governance). According to this principle, professionals have an obligation to (1) recognize a person's capacities and perspectives and right to make choices and (2) treat that person so as to allow them to act autonomously. The second principle, *non-maleficence*, is the principle concerned with the obligation not to inflict harm or expose people to unnecessary risks. It is especially relevant for the protection of people who are not competent in some way. The principle of *beneficence* is the converse of non-maleficence: the obligation to take positive steps to help others. It provides the essential justification and goal for the health professions. The final principle is *justice*, which addresses entitlements: people should receive their due and should be treated fairly. It is not to say that people should be treated equally in every way, since not all people are equally competent or equally healthy, and people who are ill have a right to greater resources.

There are also four more specific guidelines or rules concerning dentist–patient communication. The rule of *veracity* concerns the importance of telling the truth. Lying is wrong, but is not the same as non-disclosure of information. Two related rules are privacy and confidentiality, which are sometimes confused with each other. *Privacy* refers to the respect for limited access to a person, whether it be viewing, touching or obtaining information. Patients grant access to themselves when they consult a dentist, but not unlimited access. For example, there have been recent discussions on whether patients should be required to be tested for HIV before major dental surgery: a question of privacy. Patients may not agree with dentists about the amount of information they ought to divulge: one survey indicated that many patients would not tell their dentist about drug abuse or that they had a venereal disease (McDaniel et al., 1995). This may be because patients are unsure whether the information would be kept confidential. *Confidentiality* refers to the dentist's obligation to restrict access to any information provided by patients. There ought not to be any disclosure of information to others without the patient's permission or without very good reason. This applies to both communications and records. Confidentiality can be violated when there is deliberate disclosure or when there is negligence (e.g. leaving notes in a public place). The final rule, *fidelity*, concerns promise-keeping, especially for a health professional to seek a patient's welfare and not to be negligent with information. Fidelity can be problematic in the case of clinical research. Although the clinical role is primarily concerned with a patient's welfare, a research project may be primarily for society's benefit, not the patient's.

Ethical dilemmas

Ethical considerations involve the process of examining and weighing up the importance of these principles in particular situations. Sometimes there is no one 'right' answer when one principle (such as autonomy) might conflict with another (such as beneficence). For example, a patient may refuse treatment (such as a restoration) which is manifestly in their best interests. Or there may be a conflict between the rule of privacy and the principle of autonomy. Does a dentist have the right to know whether a patient is HIV positive?

Doyal and Cannell (1993) discuss the dilemma of deciding whether to inform a professional organization of another dentist's misdoings or incompetence. On the one hand, dentists have obligations to their patients. People trust their dentists to provide them with the best care possible. Breaches of this trust would undermine the dentist–patient relationship. If a dentist were acting incompetently and causing harm to patients, steps ought to be taken to stop such practice. On the other hand, dentists also have obligations to their fellow professionals. At what point do concerns about patient welfare outweigh the proper responsibilities towards a colleague, who may also be a friend? Doyal and Cannell argue that there may be many situations in which patients, rather than colleagues, should be protected.

Fluoridation of the water supply

Fluoridation of the public water supply is a good example of an ethical dilemma. The addition of one part per million of fluoride to the water supply is an effective method for reducing the incidence of caries in the general population. While it has been accepted in many cities and countries, it has been strongly resisted in others. It is useful to understand this debate in ethical, rather than strictly empirical, terms.

The arguments *for* fluoridation employ the principles of beneficence and justice. Fluoridation involves the principle of beneficence because it is an effective intervention which would reduce not only the number of new caries but also the number of restorations. According to the principle of beneficence, dentists have an obligation to argue for fluoridation because of its benefits to the members of society. These benefits might be the greatest for those who are most vulnerable to the development of caries. The principle of justice can also be used in the debate. The financial cost of dental restorations to society is considerable. Scarce and important resources are being used to repair damage to teeth which could be avoided simply and cheaply. Since fluoridation is less costly to society than restorations, the money saved could be used to help people in other ways, such as improved public housing or reducing unemployment. Thus, according to the principle of justice, the water supply ought to be fluoridated so that resources could be used in the most appropriate way.

However, there are ethical arguments *against* fluoridation as well. The principle of non-maleficence, which states that health professionals should not harm their patients in any way, would be violated if the addition of fluoride could have detrimental effects on patients. Those who argue against fluoridation contend that not only is there the possibility of staining of the teeth for some patients, but that the long-term consequences of adding fluoride are not yet known. There may, indeed, be some severe side-effects which might occur in the future. However, perhaps the strongest argument against fluoridation comes from those who say that it violates the right of self-determination: the principle of autonomy. According to this principle, people should not be forced to ingest a substance – in this case fluoride – against their will. Although it is possible for someone to treat their own water supply to remove fluoride in the private home, they would have no control over the presence of fluoride in water outside the home, such as in commercial beverages. In some cities, fluoride has been added to the water supply despite the protests of a minority of local citizens. When the principle of autonomy is overridden by the principle of beneficence, as it has been in such instances, *paternalism* occurs.

Informed consent

In another paper, Doyal and Cannell (1995) discuss the importance of obtaining informed consent from patients before embarking on treatment. They point out that, based on the principle of autonomy, patients have the right to decide to give or withhold their consent to treatment. Traditionally, patients trusted the dentist to decide what was best for them, but more recently this has changed, with many more people exercising their right to know, understand and consent to their treatment. It appears that patients are often unaware of the risks of treatments, and dentists, though aware themselves, do not communicate these risks (McComb et al., 1996). There are also legal issues. It is illegal for one person to touch another without his or her consent. This runs the risk of a civil action for battery. It is also possible for a dentist to be sued for negligence if he or she does not provide sufficient information about the significant hazards associated with a procedure.

There are five basic elements of consent:

1. The patient should be given sufficient information about the procedure, and the potential risks and benefits which might result. The problem here is in knowing how much detail to give.
2. The patient should be able to understand the information given. Sometimes, the information, although provided, is worded in such a technical way that understanding is difficult.
3. The patient should give his or her consent voluntarily, without coercion of any kind.
4. The patient needs to be competent to give a decision. At what age is a child competent to agree to a procedure and, perhaps more problematically, at what age is a child competent to refuse?
5. Finally, the patient needs to provide verbal or written consent. Usually, verbal consent is adequate for most routine procedures in dentistry, but written consent is needed for more invasive or dangerous procedures.

Summary

While most research relating psychology to dentistry has concerned patients, the personal qualities and behaviour of the dentist are also significant.

Communication involves both verbal and non-verbal behaviour. While coercion, coaxing and belittling patients increases disruptions, explanation and direction serve to increase cooperation. The words spoken by a dentist are embedded within a large number of non-verbal signals, such as eye gaze, proximity and gestures. These non-verbal signs have a strong influence on the meaning of verbal messages. They, too, can affect cooperation: for example, gently patting a patient can reduce fearful behaviour while restraint seems to increase it.

One of the more important personal qualities needed by health care professionals is called 'accurate empathy', which involves both the ability to understand what patients mean by their verbal and non-verbal communication and the ability to express this understanding to them. Some dental schools include training programmes in their curricula which are designed to improve these abilities, sometimes through direct instruction and sometimes by observation of students' behaviour with patients.

There are many ethical issues and dilemmas in dentistry. Currently, patients' rights to autonomy – especially to decide what types of treatment they will receive – is a crucial aspects of dental care.

Practice implications

- Encouraging patients to make their own decisions about treatment options can often increase satisfaction and reduce complaints.
- Making tape-recordings of consultations (with the consent of patients and other staff) and reviewing these with colleagues is a powerful way of increasing social skills.
- Every interaction between a dentist and patient has ethical implications.

Suggested reading

For an overview of ethical philosophy, see Beauchamp, T. and Childress, J. (1994). *Principles of Biomedical Ethics*. Oxford: Oxford University Press and for specific guidelines, the British Dental Association (1993). *Ethical and Legal Obligations of Dental Practitioners*. London: BDA.

References

Argyle, M. and Ingram, R. (1972). Gaze, mutual gaze and proximity. *Semiotica*, 6, 32–44.
Byrne, P. and Heath, C. (1980). Practitioner's use of non-verbal behaviour in real consultations. *J. R. Coll. Gen. Pract.*, 30, 327–331.
DiMatteo, M. and DiNicola, D. (1982). *Achieving Patient Compliance*. Oxford: Pergamon.
Doyal, L. and Cannell, H. (1993). Whistleblowing: the ethics of revealing professional incompetence within dentistry. *Br. Dent. J.*, 174, 95–101.
Doyal, L. and Cannell, H. (1995). Informed consent and the practice of good dentistry. *Br. Dent. J.*, 178, 454–460.
Furnham, A. (1983). Social skills and dentistry. *Br. Dent. J.*, 154, 404–408.
Gershen, J. A., Marcus, M., Strohlein, A., et al. (1980). An application of interpersonal process recall for teaching behavioural science in dentistry. *J. Dent. Educ.*, 44, 268–269.
Hall, E. (1967). *The Hidden Dimension*. London: Bodley Head.
Hasegawa, T., Lange, B., Bower, C. and Purtilo, R. (1988). Ethical or legal perceptions by dental practitioners. *J. Am. Dent. Assoc.*, 116, 354–360.
Hirsch, B., Levine, B. and Tiber, N. (1973). Effects of dentist authoritarianism on patient evaluation of dentures. *J. Prosthet. Dent.*, 30, 745–748.

Jackson, E. (1975). Establishing rapport. 1. Verbal interaction. *J. Oral Med.*, **30**, 105–110.

Jackson, E. (1978). Convergent evidence for the effectiveness of interpersonal skill training for dental students. *J. Dent. Educ.*, **42**, 517–523.

Kress, G., Hasegawa, T. and Guo, I. (1995). A survey of ethical dilemmas and practical problems encountered by practicing dentists. *J. Am. Dent. Assoc.*, **126**, 1554–1561.

Lefer, L., Pleasure, M. and Rosenthal, L. (1962). A psychiatric approach to the denture patient. *Psychosom. Res.*, **6**, 199–207.

Levy, R., Domoto, P., Olson, D., et al. (1980). Evaluation of one-to-one behavioural training. *J. Dent. Educ.*, **44**, 221–222.

McDaniel, T., Miller, D., Jones, R. and Davis, M. (1995). Assessing patient willingness to reveal health history information. *J. Am. Dent. Assoc.*, **126**, 375–379.

McComb, J., Wright, J, Fox, N. and O'Brien, K. (1996). Perceptions of the risks and benefits of orthodontic treatment. *Community Dent. Health*, **13**, 133–138.

Melamed, B., Bennett, C., Jerrell, G., et al. (1983). Dentists' behavior management as it affects compliance and fear in pediatric patients. *J. Am. Dent. Assoc.*, **196**, 324–330.

Osborne, B. (1993). Confidentiality – at any price? *Br. Dent. J.*, **175**, 350–351.

Rutzen, S. (1973). The social importance of orthodontic rehabilitation: report of a five-year follow-up study. *J. Health Soc. Behav.*, **14**, 233–240.

Sfikas, J. (1996). Guarding the files. *J. Am. Dent. Assoc.*, **127**, 1248–1252.

Szasz, T. and Hollender, M. (1956). A contribution to the philosophy of medicine the basic models of the doctor–patient relationship. *Arch. Intern. Med.*, **97**, 585–592.

Weinstein, P., Getz, T., Ratener, P., et al. (1982). The effect of dentists' behaviors on fear-related behaviors in children. *J. Am. Dent. Assoc.*, **104**, 32–38.

Weinstein, P. and Nathan, J. (1988). The challenge of fearful and phobic children. *Den. Clin. North Am.*, **32**, 667–692.

Wurster, C., Weinstein, P. and Cohen, A. (1979). Communication patterns and pedodontics. *Percept. Mot. Skills*, **48**, 159–166.

Index

Printed in the United Kingdom
by Lightning Source UK Ltd.
130262UK00001B/121-123/A

9 780723 610571